MEDICAL ETHICS 101

KHAN'S CASES

Please visit www.myERdoctor.com to contact the author, view citations, and experience other amazing things.

Great for USMLE™ prep!

The 101 Cases that you MUST KNOW

Featuring the most up to date practice questions with answers and explanations

Real-world scenarios for every student, resident, and practicing physician

By: Maryam Arshad, MD and Sajid Khan, MD
USMLE is a registered trademark of the Federation of State Medical Boards (FSMB) and the National Board of Medical Examiners (NBME), neither of which endorses or sponsors this product.

© Copyright 2017, Createspace

The text of this publication, or any part of it, may not be reproduced without written permission from the author or publisher. All rights reserved. Photocopying or illegal distribution of any of this text is forbidden and violators may be prosecuted. No part of this publication may be stored in a database or retrieval system without permission from the author.

The authors and publishers have provided this text to offer accurate information with regard to the subject matters covered. If legal advice or other expert assistance is required, please consult with an attorney. The authors and publishers hereby waive any and all legal responsibility for any action taken as a result of this text.

"A man without ethics is a wild beast loosed upon this world"

- Albert Camus

Ethical situations are almost never black or white. There are a number of legal principles (autonomy, beneficence, substituted judgment, end-of-life issues, abortion, etc) which play a significant role in the practice of medicine that can help form a basis for decision-making. The American Medical Association's 'Code of Medical Ethics' also offers guidelines to form reasonable approaches to such subjective cases. Ethical issues will arise during examinations: all of the questions presented here are questions that are very likely to appear on the boards and all are scenarios that any physician can encounter in real life. Topics have been arranged in random order to emulate testing conditions – if you would like to see them organized by topic, please refer to the index at the end.

We sincerely hope you enjoy this book and that it helps bring you some measure of success in the future.

Medical Ethics 101

Case:

A 40 year old male comes your office because he has been 'feeling bad lately'. He says that for the past three months he has been having trouble sleeping and has not had the desire to go out. He has stopped going to baseball games with friends, which had been something he enjoyed. He is obese and notes that while most of his friends are married and have children, he has difficulty getting a date. He feels worthless and has even missed days at work as he finds it difficult to concentrate. The most important question to ask is:

A) "Have you had any recent stressors in your life?"

B) "Do you ever feel like life is not worth living?"

C) "Do you think that your life would be much better if you were dating?"

D) "I'm having some friends over to watch the baseball game tonight – would you like to come?"

E) "Have you tried losing weight? I would be happy to advise you on diet and exercise habits...."

Medical Ethics 101

Answer:

B) "Do you ever feel like life is not worth living?"

Explanation:

SIG E CAPS

Screening for major depression is important. An easy way to remember the diagnostic criteria is SIG E CAPS:

S – sleep disturbances
I – interest decreased in activities
G- guilt or worthlessness
E – energy decreased
C – concentration difficulties
A – appetite disturbances
P – psychomotor retardation/agitation
S – suicidal thoughts

Having a depressed mood and at least four of the above for at least two weeks meets the criteria for major depression[1].

This patient has symptoms suggestive of major depressive disorder, and it is important to assess whether or not he is suicidal. Identifying the source of his depression is important, and stressors (be they related to work, finances, relationships, etc) are essential to identify in order to treat the underlying cause. Avoid forming relationships with your patient outside of the professional setting as that can lead you to make decisions that might not always be in the best interest of the patient – in other words, your relationship might influence how you treat him. While obesity is associated with many serious medical conditions, his depression may lead him to commit suicide.

Medical Ethics 101

Case:

A 4 year old girl is brought to the ER after falling off a swing. She appears to have a fractured right forearm. Sensation and pulses are intact. She is accompanied by her 18 year old babysitter. Both the babysitter and emergency room staff are unable to contact her parents for consent to treat. What is the most appropriate response?

A) Continue attempts to contact the parents to obtain consent

B) Obtain an x-ray and treat the fracture appropriately

C) Obtain consent from the babysitter as she has assumed responsibility in this case

D) Using implied consent, reduce the fracture as you continue attempts to contact the parents

Medical Ethics 101

Answer:

A) Continue attempts to contact the parents to obtain consent

Explanation:

The vignette implies that the fracture is *not* life or limb-threatening. In such cases, you need to make reasonable attempts to obtain consent from parents or legal guardians[2]. Babysitters have no more of a legal right to make decisions than do strangers. There is no indication in the question that fracture reduction is necessary – in fact no mention is made of a deformity and the extremity has no neurovascular deficits so it would be inappropriate to reduce the fracture without 1: an x-ray and 2: consent.

Medical Ethics 101

Case:

You are in clinic seeing a patient for routine followup. The patient has a history of schizophrenia and informs you that he doesn't like his boss. The patient asks if everything he tells you is confidential. You confirm that it is and he admits, "sometimes I think I might kill him if I get the chance." What is the most appropriate action?

A) Maintain confidentiality while attempting to discourage the patient from his plan

B) Inform law enforcement agencies of the threat to the patient's boss

C) Inform the patient's boss of the threat

D) Inform both the patient's boss and law enforcement of the threat

E) Admit the patient for homicidal ideations but maintain confidentiality

Medical Ethics 101

Answer:

D) Inform both the patient's boss and law enforcement of the threat

Explanation:

'Duty to warn' requires a clinician who has reasonable grounds to believe that a client may be in imminent danger of harming others to warn the possible victims. **'Duty to warn' is one of the few exceptions to a patient's right to confidentiality.** In cases of suicidality and homicidality, you have a moral and legal obligation to inform the potential victim and the proper authorities. If law enforcement is informed and the potential victim is not informed then you are held liable if there is injury to the victim. It will be necessary to admit the patient for homicidal ideations, so that he can receive proper psychiatric treatment – but the police and the person at risk should still be warned.

Tarasoff v Regents of the University of California:
Tatiana Tarasoff was murdered by Prosenjit Poddar, who had received psychological services in the university counseling center. Poddar informed his psychologist that he wanted to kill Tarasoff, and following the session his psychologist informed the campus police. The psychologist also wrote a letter requesting assistance to the chief of campus police. Poddar was briefly detained by police and questioned, then released because his mental state seemed stable. No one ever warned Tatiana Tarasoff and Poddar eventually killed Tarasoff. The case was settled out of court but established the precedence of 'duty to warn'.

Jablonski by Pahls v United States:
Extended a clinician's responsibility even further, concluding that duty to warn also entails reviewing previous records, which may contain history of previous violent behavior and therefore be a predictor of future violence. These laws vary from state to state, and at least four states have still not adopted a 'duty to warn' approach[3,4].

Medical Ethics 101

Case:

A 30 year old pregnant woman presents to your clinic for prenatal care. She has a history of having had syphilis in the past and chlamydia earlier in this pregnancy. She has never had an HIV test done. She is 36 weeks gestation and is offered an HIV test as part of her prenatal care – but declines to have it done. Despite your best attempts at discussing the importance of early detection and the risk to her unborn child, she continues to refuse. What is your response?

A) Do not perform the test as she has the right to refuse

B) Perform the test, as it is necessary to protect the health of the baby

C) Administer empiric antitretroviral therapy to prevent perinatal transmission

D) Obtain consent from the father of the child

E) Obtain a court order to test the patient

Medical Ethics 101

Answer:

A) Do not perform the test as she has the right to refuse

Explanation:

An unborn child does not have the same rights as an individual under the law. Therefore, mandating that the patient undergo the test for the sake of her unborn child falls flat. Pregnant women may opt-out from HIV testing, in which case the physician should continue attempts to educate the patient and encourage testing, but cannot force it upon her[5]. Furthermore, HIV testing typically requires an additional layer of consent.

In October 2012, a woman in New York sued her physician for informing her that she was HIV positive – she claims she never consented for the test[6]. Testing patients against their will or without their knowledge is acceptable only in cases where you are trying to prevent harm to another person. Since the law does not recognize the unborn, the mother's health and decisions take priority.

Medical Ethics 101

Case:

A 60 year old male presents to the emergency room with shortness of breath. He has a history of diabetes, HTN, and coronary artery disease. His labs confirm that he is in acute renal failure with a potassium of 7 and will need dialysis. While reviewing his chart, you find a DNR/DNI (do not resuscitate/do not intubate) form that he has filled out. He confirms that he still feels the same way and would like both the DNR and DNI forms to be kept on the front of his chart. Which of the following is most appropriate?

A) Inform the patient that you cannot admit him to the hospital if the DNR/DNI forms remain active

B) Ask the patient if he has a durable power of attorney or surrogate decision maker that he would like you to consult

C) Dialyze the patient anyway and admit him to the ICU, but do not intubate him if it becomes necessary

D) Treat the patient with medications only and admit him to a medical floor bed

Medical Ethics 101

Answer:

C) Dialyze the patient anyway and admit him to the ICU, but do not intubate him if it becomes necessary

Explanation:

Patients with a DNR form can still be treated and admitted to an intensive care unit. A DNR order is designed to keep the patient from receiving cardiopulmonary resuscitation (eg defibrillation, antiarrythmics, CPR). Hyperkalemia in this case is life-threatening; withholding this treatment is inappropriate and independent of a DNR order[7,8]. Identifying a surrogate decision maker in this case is unnecessary as there is no reason to suspect that the patient cannot make decisions on his own. Do not confuse DNR orders with palliative care – there is no reason the patient should not be admitted to the intensive care unit.

Medical Ethics 101

Case:

You are the inpatient physician taking care of an elderly woman who will likely be diagnosed with metastatic cancer pending the results of a biopsy. Although the patient is alert and oriented, she is very sick and the family has concerns regarding lack of a cure. The family asks that you inform them first about the results of the biopsy. They do not want to upset the patient further. What should you tell them?

A) You will communicate the results to them first

B) You ask for the ethics committee to get involved

C) Tell them that you are obligated to inform the patient of the findings

D) Explain to them that that decision can only be made by the healthcare proxy

Medical Ethics 101

Answer:

C) Tell them that you are obligated to inform the patient of the findings

Explanation:

Your first duty is to keep the patient fully informed.

'Therapeutic privilege' grants you the right to withhold information from a patient if you believe that he or she will suffer **serious psychological harm** from possessing that information[9-11]. Unless there is significant evidence that the patient would become suicidal or otherwise mentally unstable, you have a duty to the patient first, not the family. In such cases it is always best to have a conversation with both the patient and the family prior to testing, so that expectations can be conveyed and open discussions can be had.

A health-care proxy's participation is only necessary if the patient loses decision-making capacity. So long as the patient is awake and has capacity to make decisions for themselves, they should do so – not a durable power of attorney, not a surrogate decision maker, and not a health-care proxy. Ethics committees typically only need to get involved if, for whatever reason, a patient is not able to make a decision, the family cannot agree on a decision, *and* the physician is unsure of what is in the patient's best interests.

Medical Ethics 101

Case:

A 35 year old male presents to your office for a first-time visit. His past medical history includes a diagnosis of epilepsy for which he takes medication. He has been seizure-free for six months, and confides that he has just gotten a job as a bus driver. He has had difficulty finding employment and understands that he shouldn't be driving, but states that since he has not had a seizure for six months he thinks he should be okay. How should you respond?

A) Advise him to disclose this to his employer. If he does not, then give him strict precautions on when to stop driving and when to return to your office.

B) Since he has been seizure-free for six months, it is permissible for him to drive.

C) Advise him to disclose this to his employer. If he does not, then report him to the DMV.

D) Advise him to disclose this to his employer. Make him sign a written form indicating that you have informed him of all of the risks so that you are not liable in case of an accident.

Medical Ethics 101

Answer:

C) Advise him to disclose this to his employer. If he does not, then report him to the DMV.

Explanation:

Driving restrictions for persons with seizure disorders are designed to protect the public safety. Situations such as these will require a delicate balance between maintaining patient confidentiality and protecting the community. The best initial course of action is to have an open discussion with the patient – verbalize understanding of his situation, explain your rationale, and make sure he is aware of all of the potential risks. Advise him to discuss the situation with his employer and disclose his medical history. Violating confidentiality will carry with it serious consequences, and can limit a physician's effectiveness in establishing a rapport with his or her patients. Therefore, this conversation should be had early and with full disclosure of what might happen if a patient does not handle the situation appropriately.

The majority of states recommend voluntary physician reporting; a few states have mandatory reporting laws (Nevada, Delaware, and New Jersey require reporting for epilepsy). Failure to report may lead to physician liability if the patient as a driver is involved in an accident[12-16].

According to the American Medical Association (AMA): "In those situations where clear evidence of substantial driving impairment implies a strong threat to patient and public safety, and where physicians' advice to discontinue driving privileges is disregarded, physicians have an ethical duty to notify the DMV of the medical conditions which would impair safe driving. This duty exists even when reporting impaired drivers is not mandated by law. Departments of Motor Vehicles should be the final determiners of the inability to drive safely."

Medical Ethics 101

Case:

A patient was involved in a serious motor vehicle accident. After two weeks of being in the ICU, the patient is finally declared brain dead. You are the ICU resident who has cared for the patient throughout his stay, and have formed the closest relationship with his family. Who should obtain consent for organ donation?

A) You

B) Your attending

C) Organ procurement coordinator / Organ donor network

D) Social worker

Medical Ethics 101

Answer:

C) Organ procurement coordinator / Organ donor network

Explanation:

The individuals who diagnose and treat a patient's condition should be clearly distinguishable from those who pursue organ procurement and transplantation. If the physician, who is supposed to be providing optimum medical care and treating a patient to the best of his or her ability, is at the same time requesting consent to harvest organs, it can give conflicting perceptions to the family. According to the US Dept of Health and Human Services, a hospital will notify its local organ procurement organization of every patient that has died or is nearing death – and the procurement coordinator will seek consent from the next of kin[17,18].

Medical Ethics 101

Case:

A 30 year old nurse was drawing blood on a patient and accidentally stuck herself with a needle that had several drops of the patient's blood on it. The patient is admitted for an abscess in his antecubital area and is a known IV drug abuser. His HIV status is unknown. What should the physician caring for the nurse do at this point?

A) Request consent from the patient for an HIV test. If he refuses, you cannot draw blood.

B) Review the patient's chart to first find out if he has ever had a test. If not, request consent from the patient.

C) Reassure the nurse that the likelihood of contracting HIV from a needle stick is extremely low and that she will need to keep follow up with occupational health for serial blood draws to make sure she doesn't sero-convert.

Medical Ethics 101

Answer:

A) Request consent from the patient for an HIV test. If he refuses, you cannot draw blood.

Explanation:

If the patient is HIV-positive, promptly treating the nurse will greatly reduce her chance of becoming HIV-positive and increase her life span should she end up sero-converting. While the likelihood of contracting the disease may be low, that does not permit forgoing the test. Reviewing the patient's chart is technically a violation of patient confidentiality as your intentions are not to help the patient in any way. Furthermore, discovering a previous negative result does not absolve you of the duty to perform an HIV test.

This is a gray area of medical ethics as the need to protect the healthcare provider must be weighed against the need to protect a patient's autonomy. Laws vary from state to state; 36 states have laws that allow unconsented HIV testing of source patients. For the purposes of a test, however, conditions are always ideal and patient rights are always upheld.

If a patient refuses to have blood drawn for an HIV test, a thorough explanation of risks and benefits should be made. If the source patient continues to refuse to consent to HIV testing, obtaining a court order to draw additional blood may be necessary[20].

Jane Doe v Yale University School of Medicine:
In 1988 a first year intern was asked to place an arterial line on an AIDS patient in the ICU. She had a needlestick exposure and contracted HIV at the age of 25. She sued the university for inadequate training. She argued that she had only done the procedure once before and had only received a total of ten minutes of training on universal precautions to prevent HIV infection. She was awarded $12.2 million[21].

Medical Ethics 101

Case:

A 16 year old girl presents to your office with a chief complaint of burning with urination. She admits that she is sexually active and does not always use protection. Her urinalysis is negative. She has never had a pelvic exam before but you decide that would be the next most appropriate step. She consents to the exam but asks that you not tell her parents she has had one done. What is the next most appropriate step?

A) Advise the patient that you will have to inform her parents. If she refuses, you cannot do the pelvic exam without their consent

B) Inform the patient that one parent will need to be present for the exam

C) Inform the patient that if she has a sexually transmitted infection, you will not contact her parents. However, if the exam is negative you will need to tell them why she was seen in your office

D) Do not inform her parents and proceed with the exam

Medical Ethics 101

Answer:

D) Do not inform her parents and proceed with the exam

Explanation:

Minors have a right to access sexual healthcare without the consent or notification of their parents. They may be checked for sexually transmitted infections or started on birth control without the physician contacting their parents. Communication with parents should always be encouraged, and in this case in particular the physician should have an open discussion with the patient about her relationship with her parents. In the end, if the adolescent, regardless of age, demands confidentiality, then legally you must comply. By the same token, a parent cannot demand that their daughter undergo a pelvic examination without the patient's consent.

Medical Ethics 101

Case:

A patient presents to the ER unresponsive. His wife reports that he had a headache last night and she found him this way this morning. CT scan reveals a large intracranial bleed. After a thorough exam and appropriate consultations, he is declared brain dead. His driver's license indicates that he is to be an organ donor, and you see a heart shaped symbol on his license - but his wife is very emotional and does not want his organs removed. She is certain he would not have wanted them taken. What is the most appropriate course of action?

A) Inform the wife that since he registered as an organ donor, you will respect his wishes

B) Attempt to answer all of the wife's concerns and obtain her consent, but if you are not able to, do not proceed

C) Obtain an ethics consult

D) Have the wife speak to an organ procurement coordinator to obtain consent – if they are unable to then do not remove his organs

Medical Ethics 101

Answer:

A) Inform the wife that since he registered as an organ donor, you will respect his wishes

Explanation:

Laws governing such a case vary from state to state. Until 2007, there was no official record of people who wanted to be donors. The Department of Safety driver's license and ID card application and renewal forms now include the statement: "Yes, I want to be an organ and tissue donor." Checking 'yes' on the form automatically enrolls the applicant in the Donate Life Registry, and a small heart-shaped symbol will be printed on the applicant's driver license or ID card at the top right of the picture. A signed and witnessed donor card (or back of the driver's license) does grant authorization for organ and/or tissue recovery. By registering, your desire to donate is stored in a secure, confidential database. Should your death result in the opportunity for you to be a donor, an official record of your donor designation will be readily available and cannot be overturned by your family.

If the patient had signed up before 2007, you would need to check to verify his registration as a donor. If he signed up as a donor on his license before 2007, but never registered with the national organ donor registry, his wife/family has the right to overturn his decision. For the most part, as long as a signed donor card or license is present, you should abide by it. Even when a patient has a signed organ donation card, the organ procurement coordinator still often seeks family permission to proceed with donation. The Uniform Anatomical Gift Act established that a properly signed document will be honored over any familial objections[29]. In the United States, however, it is customary to request permission from the next-of-kin. This is a difficult question to answer correctly, as the true legal answer can vary from state to state and depends on when the question was written. To summarize, if the patient is registered or has a heart-shaped symbol on their license, they have made it clear that they wishes to donate their organs[22-26].

Medical Ethics 101

Case:

An 80 year old male is brought to the emergency department after a syncopal event. You see in his chart that he has a history of metastatic lung cancer and recently completed chemotherapy. He is hypoxic and has waxing/waning consciousness. The decision is made to intubate the patient as he is not able to protect his airway and will likely go into cardiac arrest without the assisted ventilation. He is successfully intubated and thirty minutes later his grandson arrives with an advance directive indicating that he does not wish to be intubated. The son thinks his father may have changed his mind since the directive was signed. Which of the following is the most appropriate step?

A) Extubate the patient and provide supportive care

B) Obtain a court order to maintain the intubation

C) Utilizing substituted judgment, maintain the intubation

D) Maintain the intubation until you've had a chance to speak with his family

Medical Ethics 101

Answer:

D) Maintain the intubation until you've have a chance to speak with his family

Explanation:

Although the patient has made his wishes clear, families can often provide insight into whether or not the patient would have actually wanted to maintain his DNI order. For instance, he may have recently responded well to chemotherapy and had a sudden change in health that has made him want to prolong his life, and has communicated this to his family, but has not yet reflected it in his official end-of-life documents. To extubate and allow him to die would preclude this discussion from ever taking place – it would be most appropriate to gather the family and allow them to verify that this is what he would have wanted.

Studies have shown that in patients who die from cardiac arrest, family members who are brought to the bedside during cardiac resuscitation have lower rates of depression and anxiety[27]. Family involvement can never be understated. While it is inappropriate to supersede an advance directive, in this case the directive was not known about beforehand – in no way should you automatically withdraw the tube and allow the patient to die without speaking to his family.

Medical Ethics 101

Case:

You are seeing patients in the emergency department when two police officers arrive and show you their proper identification. The identification is legitimate. The officers inform you that they are performing an investigation into one of your patients on charges of driving under the influence of alcohol. The patient is in the ER following a motor vehicle accident. They ask if you checked a blood alcohol level, which you *did* as part of the routine workup, and they ask if it was above the legal driving limit of 0.8, which it was. What should you do?

A) Give them the results, since the patient broke the law by drinking with an alcohol level above the legal limit

B) Ask them to sign a release for the chart

C) Tell them you cannot show them the chart unless there is a signed release from the patient

D) Tell the nurse who is caring for the patient what the results were, out loud, so that they can hear yet you are not violating confidentiality

Medical Ethics 101

Answer:

C) Tell them you cannot show them the chart unless there is a signed release from the patient

Explanation:

You cannot release a patient's medical records unless there is a signed release from the patient or there is a court order, warrant, or subpoena. This is true no matter who is asking. All information contained in a patient's chart should be considered the property of the patient[28]. While you may morally disagree with not informing the police about someone who was driving while intoxicated, you cannot legally inform anyone outside of the patient.

It *is* permitted to violate confidentiality in order to protect the health or well-being of a third party, such as when a patient does not disclose a history of HIV or tuberculosis to others. In such cases the AMA has advised that physicians should, within the constraints of the law, attempt to persuade the infected patient to cease endangering the third party. If persuasion fails notify authorities, and if authorities take no action then notify the third party[29,30].

Medical Ethics 101

Case:

A 60 year old patient with lung cancer develops respiratory failure and is intubated. He previously named his best friend as durable power of attorney. His friend believes the patient would have wanted his life support withdrawn based on a recent conversation about test results. However, the patient had also made a living will stipulating that all measures should be undertaken to maintain his life. The patient's son believes his father's living will reflects his wishes and wants everything done to maintain his life. What should you do?

A) Appoint the son as durable power of attorney since he is the next of kin, and follow his wishes

B) Keep the patient on life support in accordance with the patient's living will

C) Respect the decision of the durable power of attorney and withdraw life support

D) Use 'substituted judgment' to determine what the patient would have wanted in such a case

Medical Ethics 101

Answer:

C) Respect the decision of the durable power of attorney and withdraw life support

Explanation:

This is truly a gray area of medical ethics. So much so that Kaplan™ states a durable power of attorney can override a living will while UWorld™ claims the opposite. The majority consensus is that the appointed durable power of attorney supersedes even a living will[31]. The patient, in good state of mind, believed that his friend would make decisions with which he would agree. It is always appropriate to facilitate a discussion between people involved in making end of life decisions, but it is unethical to try to make the choice. In the rare circumstance when there are two conflicting documents then the more recent document will offset the previous one. Circumstances may have changed since the patient made his living will (he could have been diagnosed with metastatic disease for instance) – therefore the durable power of attorney carries the responsibility of making the decision that he thinks best fits what the patient would have made given the current situation.

Medical Ethics 101

Case:

A patient was driving on an expired driver's license when he is involved in a fatal car accident. According to his license he wished to be an organ donor. Family cannot be reached and you must make a decision of whether or not to allow the harvesting of his organs as this is a time-sensitive decision. What should you do?

A) Accept the organs as the patient had expressed his wishes

B) Decline him as an organ donor candidate as his signed consent (driver's license) has expired

C) Accept the organs using the 'substituted judgment' standard

Medical Ethics 101

Answer:

B) Decline him as an organ donor candidate as his signed consent has expired

Explanation:

In cases where you have to make a time-sensitive decision and don't have the luxury of continuing attempts to contact family members, you should treat the license as a consent form. And any form that has expired is no longer valid. Substituted judgment has no place here – you can never remove organs from a patient without consent from either the patient or his next of kin.

Medical Ethics 101

Case:

A 35 year old female who is 6 weeks pregnant presents to your clinic asking for referral for an abortion – she has three children already and was going to schedule a tubal ligation when she discovered she was pregnant. You agree to refer her to a specialist, but while filling out her paperwork you receive a call from her husband. He pleads with you to not refer her for an abortion, informing you that the patient has schizophrenia. The patient does not appear delusional and is not having any hallucinations, but her medical record does indicate that she carries a diagnosis of schizophrenia. What should you do?

A) Have the patient undergo a psychiatric evaluation before referring her for an abortion

B) Inform the patient that you cannot refer her for an abortion due to her medical history

C) Refer the patient for an abortion

D) Inform the patient that you cannot refer her for an abortion due to her lack of competency to make decisions

E) Ask the ethics committee for help in making a decision

Medical Ethics 101

Answer:

C) Refer the patient for an abortion

Explanation:

Having a diagnosis of schizophrenia does not automatically make one incompetent. Competency is typically determined by the legal system (usually with input from psychiatrists who can perform a competency assessment[32,33]). Capacity, on the other hand, is what a patient must possess in order to make medical decisions for themselves. There is nothing in this question to suggest that the patient lacks capacity. Patients with psychiatric diagnoses still have a legal right to make decisions for themselves. The patient has a right to autonomy – she has not made any statements which should raise suspicion.

Medical Ethics 101

Case:

A 12 year old child and his mother are involved in a serious motor vehicle accident. The child is found to have a liver laceration and is hypotensive. The mother has a pelvic fracture and also appears to have internal bleeding. Both will require blood transfusion to survive. The husband rushes into the emergency department and presents cards indicating that each member of the family is a Jehovah's witness and that it is against their religion to accept blood. What should you do?

A) Given that this is a life threatening emergency, transfuse both patients as needed

B) Transfuse the child but not the mother

C) Transfuse the mother but not the child

D) Respect the religious wishes and do not transfuse either patient

Medical Ethics 101

Answer:

B) Transfuse the child but not the mother

Explanation:

State v. Perricone: Denying medical care to a child is not within the parents' First Amendment right of freedom of religion: "The right to practice religion freely does not include the liberty to expose...a child...to ill health or death. Parents may be free to become martyrs themselves. But it does not follow that they are free...to make martyrs of their children..."[34,35]

Therefore, in life threatening situations, persons over the age of eighteen can make a choice and the physician must abide by it (so long as the person has capacity to make decisions). In emergency cases where a person is unresponsive or consent cannot be obtained, 'implied consent' allows physicians to treat accordingly. With regard to minors, the legal guardian may withhold treatment so long as the decision is not life or limb-threatening.

Note that the answer choice might include the option to call a parent to obtain consent in case of a life-threatening injury to a child. In such cases this is still the wrong answer as consent is unnecessary and will only delay care.

Medical Ethics 101

Case:

A 45-year-old woman is brought to the hospital by her husband. The patient complains of severe abdominal pain and has right lower quadrant tenderness. She is taken to the operating room with a presumptive diagnosis of appendicitis. Surgery reveals that the appendix is normal and without inflammation. However, you notice a large tumor attached to the patient's right ovary. At this point what is the best next course of action?

A) End the surgery

B) Excise as much of the tumor as possible without coming into contact with the ovary

C) Exercising 'standard of care', remove the patient's ovary to eliminate the tumor

D) Seek consent from the patient's husband, who is sitting in the waiting room

E) Talk with the patient's husband, who is in the waiting room, about how his wife would probably want to proceed and use 'substituted judgment'

Medical Ethics 101

Answer:

A) End the surgery

Explanation:

A competent patient has the right to make all treatment decisions for themselves, including refusal of treatment. After the woman recovers from anesthesia, she is entitled to full informed consent including descriptions of the nature of the procedure, the purpose or rationale, the benefits, the risks, and the availability of alternatives[36]. With this information presented, the patient herself can make whatever treatment decision seems best to her. If she were in a coma of some duration, then we might ask the husband under the doctrine of 'substituted judgment'. But in this case she can wake up and be asked directly.

If the opposite situation were true; wherein the patient was undergoing elective surgery for removal of an ovarian cyst (for instance), but an acutely inflamed appendix was discovered – the appendix could be removed as allowing it to remain could lead to perforation/sepsis. Such a case would constitute a true medical emergency and the physician would be permitted to act without first waking the patient and obtaining consent again.

Medical Ethics 101

Case:

You see a patient in clinic – she has just received news that her quantitative hCG is declining and she is likely having a spontaneous miscarriage. She starts crying, "The Lord is punishing me! The Lord is punishing me!" What is the most appropriate response?

A) "I can see that you're very upset – would you like to talk to our priest?"

B) "This is a difficult situation, but there is no reason to think you can't carry a full term pregnancy"

C) "Let's take a minute to pray together. That will help us decide where to go from here..."

D) "This is a difficult situation. I'll allow you to gather your thoughts..."

E) "This can just happen sometimes, and it's not your fault. I don't think the Lord has anything to do with this..."

Medical Ethics 101

Answer:

D) "This is a difficult situation. I'll allow you to gather your thoughts..."

Explanation:

"Silence is golden when you can't think of a good answer"
    - Muhammad Ali

Give the patient a period of silence and allow her to process the news – then offer to educate her about what happened and what her options are going forward. Don't refer her to a priest without making sure the patient understands the situation and without at least offering your condolences first. Also, refrain from offering false hope by informing her that she can have a successful pregnancy – there is no way you can credibly make that promise to a patient. It is important to find out if the patient feels she is being punished for something, so if given the choice to ask the patient *why* she feels the Lord is punishing her, that would be appropriate as well. You should reassure her that the miscarriage is through no fault of her own, but it is best to first provide her comfort.

Medical Ethics 101

Case:

A 30 year old HIV-positive woman gives birth to a healthy baby boy. The woman has received no prenatal care. Tests are performed to assess the child's HIV status and return positive. She is clearly excited about the birth and appears to be very loving – she is constantly holding the baby and kissing him on the cheek every chance that she gets. When told of the infant's HIV results, the new mother appears oblivious, and says that she will just have to "be an even better mother to help get through this." She asks for advice while breastfeeding. The physician tells her that breastfeeding is not advisable, to which she replies, "I know that breast milk is best, and my baby deserves the best." How should the physician respond?

A) "I'm glad you are taking such good care of your baby. I'll schedule an appointment with the lactation consultant."

B) "If you breastfeed your child, the courts can remove the child from your custody."

C) "If you really want what is best for your child, you will not breastfeed."

D) "Breastfeeding increases the risk of transmitting HIV to your child. You must not do it."

E) "It's great to see how happy you are – why don't we talk more about these things after you've had some rest."

F) "Let me explain. A positive test when the child is this young is not definitive. But if you breastfeed your child, you greatly increase the chances of your child contracting HIV."

Medical Ethics 101

Answer:

F) "Let me explain. A positive test when the child is this young is not definitive. But if you breastfeed your child, you greatly increase the chances of your child contracting HIV."

Explanation:

Approximately 25% of untreated women with HIV will transmit the virus to their baby[37]. All children of HIV-positive mothers will *test* positive at birth due to the mother's antibodies. Women who are HIV-positive should not breastfeed as that can increase the chances of congenital transmission by a significant degree. Courts do have legal precedent to remove children from the custody of mothers who insist on breast-feeding[38]. Making sure the mother knows this is essential. Your choice of words is also important. Direct commands are not the best option. Instead, explain the reasons for the recommendation in a way that makes clear the risk to the child.

Medical Ethics 101

Case:

A 30 year old woman who was diagnosed with tuberculosis gives birth to a healthy baby boy. The woman has received no prenatal care. She asks about advice while breastfeeding as she knows that is what is best for her baby. The physician tells her that breastfeeding is not advisable, to which she replies, "I know that breast milk is best, and my baby deserves the best." The physician's response should be which of the following?

A) "I'm glad you are taking your new responsibilities so seriously. I'll schedule an appointment with the lactation consultant."

B) "If you insist on breastfeeding your child, the courts can remove the child from your custody."

C) "Let me explain. If you breastfeed your child, you greatly increase the chances of your child contracting TB."

Medical Ethics 101

Answer:

C) "Let me explain. If you breastfeed your child, you greatly increase the chances of your child contracting TB."

Explanation:

There are certain situations in which a mother should refrain from breastfeeding due to potential risks to her newborn. This includes mothers who are HIV positive, are undergoing chemo or radiation therapy, have untreated active tuberculosis, or are using illicit drugs[39-41].

Medical Ethics 101

Case:

Parents bring their 15 year old daughter to the emergency department. They are suspicious that she has been sexually active with her 16 year old boyfriend, and request that you do a pelvic exam and urine pregnancy test on her. The patient, who is in high school and still lives with her parents, doesn't say much until you ask her about doing a pelvic exam, at which point she replies, "I'd rather you didn't..." What is the most appropriate course of action?

A) Respect the minor's wishes, and defer all testing unless she consents

B) Perform the urine pregnancy test but inform the parents that you cannot do a pelvic exam without consent

C) Perform the pelvic exam but inform the parents that you cannot do the pregnancy test without consenting

D) Inform the patient that since she is still a minor, she must comply with her parents' request

Medical Ethics 101

Answer:

A) Respect the minor's wises, and defer all testing unless she consents

Explanation:

Typically, when a child refuses care (for instance a five year old who doesn't want sutures) – the parents can override and there isn't much of a dilemma. Problems arise when an adolescent refuses care. The refusal of care should be respected under the 'mature minor doctrine', as the fifteen year old is considered old enough to understand her actions. She certainly understands the nature and purpose of the examination. State law supports the minor when presenting for issues related to sexually transmitted diseases, contraception, and pregnancy[42].

<u>Mature minor doctrine</u>:
The authority to consent or refuse treatment for a minor has traditionally remained with a parent or guardian. Over the years, courts have gradually recognized that children younger than eighteen years who show maturity and competence deserve a voice in determining their course of medical treatment. A minor who is found able to understand short and long-term consequences is considered to be "mature" and thus able to provide informed consent/refusal for medical treatment. The minor is authorized to make decisions regarding his or her medical treatment as long as the following criteria are met: age > 14, capable of giving informed consent, treatment will benefit, treatment does not pose a great risk, and treatment is within established medical protocols. Although not every state has a mature minor doctrine, courts have recognized the need to look at certain case laws involving the ability of mature adolescents to make medical decisions[43].

Medical Ethics 101

Case:

A patient presents to your clinic with wrist pain. X-rays are negative; eventually you obtain an EMG which confirms a diagnosis of carpal tunnel syndrome. He will need a referral to an orthopedic surgeon for definitive care. There is a new orthopedic surgeon in town who is looking for referrals. You have met him before and know that he is adequately trained to care for your patient. He is offering $50 for each referral that you send to him. What is the most appropriate next step?

A) Refer the patient to the new physician

B) Refer the patient to the new physician but give the $50 referral bonus to the patient

C) Refer the patient to a different group of orthopedic surgeons, one that your partners traditionally use

D) Refer the patient to the new physician and accept the referral bonus, but inform the patient so that he is aware of it

Medical Ethics 101

Answer:

C) Refer the patient to a different group of orthopedic surgeons, one that your partners traditionally use

Explanation:

'Fee splitting' is the practice of sharing fees with professional colleagues in return for being sent referrals. Accepting payment for a referral is illegal and should never be tolerated. The AMA's Code of Medical Ethics states: "Payment by or to a physician solely for the referral of a patient is fee splitting and is unethical..."[44]. Financial incentives have a tendency to corrupt the medical decision-making of those providing care and violates the basic trust that is at the center of a physician-patient relationship.

Medical Ethics 101

Case:

You are seeing a patient in clinic who has been diagnosed with tuberculosis. He is an undocumented illegal immigrant. He is afraid of being deported if the Department of Health learns of his immigration status. What should you tell him?

A) "You have nothing to worry about - the Department of Health does not ask for your immigration status."

B) "As long as you remain compliant with treatment, there is no mandatory reporting to the government."

C) "I will fully treat you and make sure you are taken care of before the government looks into sending you back."

D) "It's important that you take the medications, and I'm sorry but legally I have to report this to the government."

Medical Ethics 101

Answer:

A) "You have nothing to worry about - the Department of Health does not ask for your immigration status."

Explanation:

As a physician you have an ethical duty to provide medical care to patients. Neither physicians nor the Department of Health report a person's immigration status to the government. The Department of Health does not even ask about immigration status. There is no mandatory reporting to the government either before, during, or after the treatment of tuberculosis, regardless of compliance. A noncompliant patient might be incarcerated against his will to take TB medications, but they don't specifically face deportation for health reasons.

Medical Ethics 101

Case:

A 23 year old is in a serious motor vehicle accident and is pronounced brain dead. It is unclear whether he was registered as an organ donor as his driver's license is not available and you must make a time-sensitive decision on whether or not he is a viable donor. His wife is unclear what he would have wanted, but she herself is a donor so she consents. Before anything can be done, his parents arrive and inform the doctors that they've never heard him discuss the issue of organ donation before and they would prefer that he not be made a donor. The wife has stepped out and is unavailable so you cannot get both parties together to discuss. You make every effort to try to get both parties together but cannot. What is the most appropriate course?

A) Accept the wife's consent and notify the organ donation network

B) Accept the parents' declination and do not notify the organ donation network

C) Make contact with the patient's siblings to help make a decision

Medical Ethics 101

Answer:

A) Accept the wife's consent and notify the organ donation network

Explanation:

This would be a good case for an ethics committee to be involved with, but the legal answer is to accept the wife's consent[45].

The Uniform Anatomical Gift Act (UAGA) governs organ donation for the purpose of transplantation. The UAGA has created a very specific hierarchy of who can give consent for donation.

The order of people who may provide consent:
- The donor him or herself
- Spouse
- Adult Children
- Parents
- Adult Siblings
- Adult Grandchildren

Medical Ethics 101

Case:

A 17 year old girl presents to your clinic. She is 12 weeks pregnant and would like to have an abortion. She does not want you to notify the father of her baby. What should be your response?

A) "You are too far along, so I can't, in good faith, encourage you to get an abortion"

B) "I can refer you to a specialist, but will need consent from the father as well"

C) "I can refer you to a specialist, and if you want me to maintain confidentiality from the father, I will"

Answer:

C) "I can refer you to a specialist, and if you want me to maintain confidentiality from the father, I will"

Explanation:

The legality of this issue can vary from state to state. Requiring *spousal* involvement before a woman can acquire an abortion has been interpreted as unconstitutional while parental involvement has been interpreted as constitutional. With minors, most states typically require at least one type of parental involvement – consent, notification, or both. 38 states require some type of parental involvement in a minor's decision to have an abortion – 21 states require one or both parents to consent to the procedure[47,48]. The Supreme Court has ruled that parental involvement laws (and all other abortion regulation) can legally make it more difficult for a female to acquire an abortion. But there is a threshold (spouse) beyond which the increased difficulties become unconstitutional.

Planned Parenthood of Southeastern Pennsylvania v Casey (1992): Spousal notification laws place an "undue burden" on a woman's ability to get an abortion, whereas parental involvement laws do not[49].

Medical Ethics 101

Case:

A 15 year old male comes to the clinic for his high school physical. His mother sits in the waiting room while you do the exam. Before you finish, the patient confesses that he thinks that he may be homosexual. He requests that you not tell his mother. When you finish the exam, his mother re-enters the room, and asks, "So, did you find anything? Everything a-okay??" How should you respond?

A) Inform the mother of what he has told you, and encourage discussion between the two

B) Tell her that everything is fine, but notify her later as she is the legal guardian and has a right to know. By not telling her in front of him, you maintain a strong relationship with him

C) Inform the mother that everything was fine and maintain confidentiality with the teenager

D) Encourage the adolescent to tell his mother, but if he does not, then bring it up on your own

Medical Ethics 101

Answer:

C) Inform the mother that everything was fine and maintain confidentiality with the teenager

Explanation:

The physician should not tell the boy's parents about his homosexual thoughts. He should encourage the patient to discuss his feelings with his mother, but in all areas dealing with sexual behavior, the minor has a legally protected right to confidentiality.

The truth is that many adolescents are not comfortable talking to their parents about controversial topics such as sex, drugs, peer pressure, etc. Studies show that adolescents are less likely to seek healthcare for sensitive issues if they believe that their parents will be informed[50]. Many adolescents are unaware of their right to confidentiality, therefore physicians should discuss this with both the patient and their parents at their first visit so that everyone is aware of it. Limitations with regards to confidentiality should be explained. Parents and patients need to also understand that if the adolescent poses a threat to self or others, confidentiality may be broken.

Medical Ethics 101

Case:

You are working in the emergency department when a patient comes in with a complicated laceration to his hand. You notify the orthopedic surgeon who comes down to see the patient. After examining and diagnosing him with a tendon laceration, he discovers that the patient is HIV positive. The surgeon asks that you refer him to another consultant, as he does not want to risk infecting himself by caring for this patient. Is he within his legal rights to refuse the patient?

A) Yes, so long as it is not a life-threatening situation physicians may refuse to see whomever they wish

B) Yes, while it is unethical to refuse a patient he is within his legal means

C) No, since the physician has formed a patient-physician relationship, he cannot abandon them unless it is outside his scope of practice

D) No, he is violating the principle of non-maleficence

Medical Ethics 101

Answer:

C) No, since the physician has formed a patient-physician relationship, he cannot abandon them unless it is outside his scope of practice

Explanation:

Generally speaking, you should care for all patients that you find appropriate for your level of expertise. Refusing patients on any basis – be it racial, religious, sexual orientation – will open you up to scrutiny from the judicial system, ethics committee, and your colleagues. Moreover, once a doctor-patient relationship has been established, a physician cannot refuse to treat unless something falls outside of his scope of practice. To do so could be considered abandonment – if a physician wishes to terminate a relationship with a patient (for noncompliance for instance) the patient should always be notified well ahead of time so they are able to establish care with another provider. Ending such a relationship should be done both in person and through the use of a notarized letter so that there is no question about it.

The AMA has made it very clear: "A physician may not ethically refuse to treat a patient whose condition is within the physician's current realm of competence solely because the patient is seropositive for HIV"[51].

At the same time, a physician must *voluntarily* enter a relationship with a patient and cannot be forced to accept new patients. This applies to cases in which a physician feels his clinic is overbooked or is wanting to decrease his workload so he declines new patients – so long as it is done without prejudice it is wholly acceptable.

Medical Ethics 101

Case:

You are a primary care provider at a busy urban center. One of your patients happens to be the trauma surgeon at the hospital. He has been seeing you for routine care and recently had an HIV test done after having a high-risk sexual encounter without using protection. His HIV test is positive. Who are you legally obligated to inform?

A) His insurance company

B) His patients, who might be at risk if he should cut himself during surgery

C) His supervisor (chair of the department)

D) The hospital human resources department

E) No one

Answer:

E) No one

Explanation:

Patients with HIV have a right to privacy as long as they are not putting others at risk. Universal precautions (gloves, gowns, sterile procedure) are meant to prevent infectious transmission, therefore you are not obligated to inform his patients. You have no obligation to inform his insurance or his employer.

In many European countries, including the UK and Scotland, physicians were long banned from practicing surgery or dentistry if they were known to be HIV positive. Such laws are in a constant state of flux, and in the UK just removed as recently as April 2014[52].

X v Y (1988):
An English court case concerning two doctors who had AIDS - a newspaper obtained confidential hospital records identifying the doctors. The court ruled that confidentiality of the records was more important than protecting the public from theoretical risks posed by the doctors[53].

Medical Ethics 101

Case:

A 12 year old boy is brought to the physician by his parents for a routine exam. You ask the parents to wait outside – when he is alone with you, the patient admits that he occasionally smokes cigarettes with his friends. When you initiate a discussion about smoking cessation, the patient says, "Smoking ain't a problem for me, doc..." Which of the following responses is most appropriate?

A) "At what point will smoking become a problem for you?"

B) "Did you know that smoking has many long-term health consequences?"

C) "Do your parents know you smoke?"

D) "Why don't you just quit now before it becomes a problem?"

E) "Don't you want to be able to run and play sports without getting short of breath?"

F) "Let me show you some pictures of what happens to the lungs of people who smoke."

Medical Ethics 101

Answer:

A) "At what point will smoking become a problem for you?"

Explanation:

You need to first understand what perceptions the child has about smoking. Once you have a grasp of what the child thinks about his habit, you can offer proper counsel. Discussing long-term consequences is not appropriate with adolescents, as they don't tend to think about long-term repercussions. Trying to instill fear into a patient (of any age) is never the right way to start off, and puts you at risk of losing your patient's trust. If you threaten to inform his parents now, he may not readily confess a different problem to you down the road. Inquiring about reasons for why the child started smoking is important, but is not the first step[54,55].

Medical Ethics 101

Case:

A major pharmaceutical company is enrolling subjects for a research study on new treatments for shingles. The study is a randomized double blind trial in which patients will either receive the generally accepted standard of Acyclovir, or the proposed new treatment. For each patient that a physician enrolls in the study, the patient receives $15 and the physician receives $15. Which statement best summarizes this arrangement?

A) This is permissible as long as the physician does not receive more compensation than the patient

B) This is permissible only if the physician gives all compensation to the patient

C) As long as the physician informs the patient, he or she may accept compensation

D) As long as the physician is being compensated, this is not permissible

Medical Ethics 101

Answer:

C) As long as the physician informs the patient, he or she may accept compensation

Explanation:

Potential research subjects should always be fully informed before they consent to any study. They should be made aware of any and all risks and benefits, as well as the expectations that will be placed upon them upon enrollment. Full disclosure is a requirement. The American Psychiatric Association (APA) states: "When involved in funded research, the ethical psychiatrist will advise human subjects of the funding source..."[56].

Medical Ethics 101

Case:

A 35 year old man comes to your office with a form to be filled as part of his pre-employment evaluation. He needs the form to give him a clean bill of health so that he can qualify for health insurance. The form also asks for an FAP gene test. This is in order for the company to determine which of its employees are at risk for colon cancer and may need long-term healthcare. What should your response be?

A) Perform the test and indicate the results on the form

B) Perform the test but do not share the results with the employer

C) Do not perform the test

D) Ask the patient if he wants the test done and the results reported

E) Order the test only if the patient has family members with the disease and is therefore at higher risk

Medical Ethics 101

Answer:

D) Ask the patient if he wants the test done and the results reported

Explanation:

As long as patients maintain decision-making capacity, they have a right to consent to any and all tests that are performed on them. Patients also have a right to confidentiality, and in most cases you must maintain this. The rare exception is where maintaining confidentiality either inadvertently puts others at risk or potentially may put the patient at risk.

The Genetic Information Nondiscrimination Act of 2008 (GINA) prohibits discrimination by health insurers and employers on the basis of genetic information. The law defines 'genetic information' as an individual's own genetic test, the genetic tests of family members, or knowledge that a family member has a genetic disorder.

Medical Ethics 101

Case:

A 12 year old boy was referred to a surgeon for elective repair of an inguinal hernia. It is scheduled for two months from today. The father provides consent for the surgery but the mother refuses on the grounds that she does not like the idea of her son having surgery. How should physicians proceed?

A) Do the surgery as long as one parent consents

B) Do not do the surgery since both parents need to sign consent

C) Do the surgery if the child consents

D) Obtain a court order to perform the surgery

E) Do not perform the surgery unless the hernia strangulates and it becomes medically necessary

Medical Ethics 101

Answer:

A) Do the surgery as long as one parent consents

Explanation:

Encouraging discussion between the two parents would be the best place to start. In actuality, you only need to obtain consent from one parent in order to make decisions regarding care of a child. Had this been a life-threatening situation, you would not need consent at all before beginning treatment.

Medical Ethics 101

Case:

You are seeing a 70 year old male patient with progressive glaucoma. His vision is severely impaired and is worse compared to his last visit six months ago. On multiple visits in the past you have advised him to stop driving but he has not. You suspect that he now has difficulty even reading the traffic signs. What is your responsibility toward this patient?

A) Maintain confidentiality but continue to encourage him to seek alternative modes of transportation

B) Notify the patient's family of the risk he is putting himself at by continuing to drive

C) Inform the patient that legally you must report him to the DMV

D) Rescind his driver's license

Medical Ethics 101

Answer:

C) Inform the patient that legally you must report him to the DMV

Explanation:

If the patients' visual acuity is so severely impaired that you suspect he is a danger to himself and to others, you must encourage the patient to find alternative transportation. You do not have the right to remove or suspend driving privileges. You do, however, have a duty to report a visually impaired driver to the DMV so that the DMV can make its own determination of whether the patient's license should be removed[57].

Laws can vary from state to state – physicians should be aware of their professional responsibilities for the states in which they practice. A report to the DMV may be a service to the patient as well as to the public. While restricting driving privileges is almost certainly an inconvenience, the risk of injury or death to both the patient and third parties due to a medical impairment is too great a risk to ignore. Physicians should consider the options in their jurisdictions and keep the best interests of the patient and the public in mind.

Medical Ethics 101

Case:

A 30 year old male patient wishes to raise some money to pay off his college loans. He has a nephew who lives in Canada who is in need of a kidney and willing to pay $20,000 for it. He comes to you for medical clearance. What should you tell him?

A) It is okay to accept money if the recipient truly needs the organ

B) It is never okay to accept money for the sale of your organs

C) It is okay to be reimbursed for the cost of travel and lodging, but not to make a profit off the sale of organs

D) It is okay so long as removing the organ you wish to sell does not put your life at risk

E) It is okay to donate your organs, but it must go to whoever is next on the list to receive an organ – you cannot choose who receives it

Medical Ethics 101

Answer:

C) It is okay to be reimbursed for the cost of travel and lodging, but not to make a profit off the sale of organs

Explanation:

If someone was allowed to receive cash for organs, it could create an unfair system whereby the wealthiest would received transplants before the sickest. You can donate to whomever you like – for instance, if your brother is in need of part of your kidney, you can choose to specifically donate to him rather than have him wait until his name is at the top of the list.

The wait list for each organ is formed differently, but the sickest people who are still strong enough to undergo surgery should receive the organs first. The only exception to this is with kidneys – since patients may survive on dialysis, the dispersement of kidney donations is on a first-come first-serve basis with the person who has waited the longest being on top of the list.

Steve Jobs:
Jobs needed a liver transplant – he couldn't legally pay for an organ, nor could he pay to cut the queue. Instead he signed up at multiple transplant centers throughout the country to improve his chances (health insurance often covers only one medical evaluation). In 2006, the median number of days from joining the liver waiting list to transplant was 306 nationally. In Tennessee, where Jobs ended up having the surgery, it was 46 days[58].

Mickey Mantle:
Mantle suffered from liver damage mostly as a result of a long history of alcohol consumption and eventual metastatic cancer. The average wait in the Dallas area for a liver transplant where Mantle was hospitalized was 130 days. An organ was found for him the night after he was listed, leading many to suspect he was given preferential treatment. He died two months after receiving the transplant.

Medical Ethics 101

Case:

A 70 year old diabetic woman presents to the emergency room with an infection on her foot. X-rays and blood work confirm suspicion for osteomyelitis and the orthopedic surgeon is consulted. He recommends IV antibiotics and amputation of the foot. Informed of this, the patient refuses and says, "I know I'm going to die eventually, and I don't want to be footless when I do." Despite the IV antibiotics her respiratory status starts to decline and she is intubated for airway support. Her family arrives and asks that the physician amputate her foot in order to help stop the spread of infection and potentially save her life. What is the most appropriate course of action?

A) Amputate her foot as she can no longer make decisions and her family is acting in her best interests

B) Treat her with antibiotics and supportive care, but do not amputate her foot

C) Consult the ethics committee

D) Find out if she has an advance directive or living will – and if that does not forbid amputation, only then should you proceed with surgery

Medical Ethics 101

Answer:

B) Treat her with antibiotics and supportive care, but do not amputate her foot

Explanation:

The patient made her wishes clear to you while she was able to, and there is no reason to not abide by them. Even if she had an advance directive indicating that she will consent to amputation in case of severe infection, the fact that she more recently refused such procedures will supersede the directive. A patient's right to make his or her own decisions – the principle of autonomy – is more important than substituted judgment.

Medical Ethics 101

Case:

A 6 year old girl is brought to the emergency department by her mother because of "fever and a rash". The mother is a poor historian and does not offer up much additional information – she appears withdrawn and tearful. The child does not make very much eye contact with you and looks at the floor throughout her visit. She does not engage you in conversation. The most appropriate next step is:

A) Admit the child to the hospital for evaluation and protection

B) Ask if there is anyone else in the house that is sick

C) Ask the mother and child separately what is concerning them

D) Obtain a psychiatry consult

E) Arrange for social services to visit the family at home

Medical Ethics 101

Answer:

C) Ask the mother and child separately what is concerning them

Explanation:

There are clearly other issues which need to be explored. Given the behavior of the mother and child, two things (of many) that need to be considered are domestic violence and child abuse. Each person may be afraid of openly talking about the problem in front of the other so it is best to talk to each individually. This will allow you to obtain additional information. Admitting the child to the hospital still leaves the mother vulnerable to domestic violence if that is the issue. Asking about sick contacts, while an important part of her medical history, is not the most appropriate next question. While a psychiatry consult may be necessary in the future, it is not immediately needed. If you suspect abuse, you should not send the child home with the parents under any circumstances.

Medical Ethics 101

Case:

A 40 year old woman comes to the office asking you to drug test her 15 year old son. She states that her son is normally a good student and is very interactive, but for the last three months he has become increasingly withdrawn. He spends more time in his room, his grades have dropped, and he does not spend as much time with his friends as he used to. She has confronted her son multiple times about his behavior, but he avoids talking about anything and denies using any alcohol or drugs. The mother appears genuinely concerned about her son and turns to you for help in figuring out what is wrong. How should you respond?

A) "Bring your son in to see me and we'll start by ordering a drug and alcohol test to rule those out"

B) "I can't legally test your son for any drugs without him consenting to it first"

C) "It's possible that your son may be suffering from depression and I think you should bring him in for me to talk to him"

D) "It sounds like your son may be suffering from depression – I'd like to refer you to a psychiatrist who can talk to both of you together...."

E) "The best place to start would be to setup an appointment with his principal at school to make sure there isn't something happening there that is negatively affecting him"

F) "This is normal teenage behavior, but why don't you bring him in to see me just to be sure"

Medical Ethics 101

Answer:

C) "It's possible that your son may be suffering from depression and I think you should bring him in for me to talk to him"

Explanation:

The mother is right to be concerned over her son's change in behavior. While drugs and alcohol can cause behavioral changes, so can mental illness such as depression. As part of your workup for depression, you will check an alcohol and drug test, but failing to tell the mother that you are concerned about depression is impotent. If you only mention 'alcohol and drugs' this reaffirms her suspicions and she might not bring her son back to see you, thinking she just needs to make him quit the substances he's not even using!

It is important to evaluate the patient on your own prior to referring him to a specialist. The mother should also set up an appointment with the school principal to address her concerns and find out if there is something else that she doesn't know about (perhaps the cause of his depression – whether or not he is picked on, if he has friends, reasons why his schoolwork may be suffering, etc) – but the physician should first speak with her son.

The minor should be questioned alone, ideally with the clinician sharing information about the parent's concerns. Minors often consent to drug testing, and when they do, the physician should first develop a plan for disclosure of test results to both parents and adolescent before ordering the test. For minors who refuse testing, it is rarely, if ever, appropriate to test. In cases of emergency where an adolescent is altered or unstable and you need to know about drugs that could be playing a role, 'implied consent' allows you to perform a urine drug screen, just as in any adult patient.

Medical Ethics 101

Case:

A 35 year old male presents to your clinic for the first time. He has a history of HIV, and despite not taking any medications he has a high CD4 count and low viral load (in other words it is very well controlled). He is married and confesses to you that he does not always use protection when having intercourse with his wife, and that she is unaware of his HIV status. Since his CD4 count is so good and he does not require treatment, he sometimes forgets that he even has it. What is the next step?

A) Encourage discussion between the husband and wife and strongly suggest he inform his wife of his HIV status

B) Inform the wife yourself of your patient's HIV status

C) Have the Department of Health notify his wife

D) If you can convince him to practice safe, protected sex – then there is no need for notification

Medical Ethics 101

Answer:

A) Encourage discussion between the husband and wife and strongly suggest he inform his wife of his HIV status

Explanation:

Encouraging discussion between the involved parties is the best first step. HIV is a mandatory reportable disease, and you *will* need to notify the Department of Health – but the first step is educating the patient on why it is important to inform his wife, and giving him the opportunity to do so.

Medical Ethics 101

Case:

A 55 year old patient presents to the emergency department complaining of chest pain. After obtaining an EKG, you inform the patient that he is having an ST elevation myocardial infarction (STEMI) and will need further intervention. You inform the patient that the risks of having an angiogram include development of a hematoma or coronary rupture – and describe the benefits of stopping the chest pain and providing definitive treatment of the infarction. He opts to forgo the angiogram because of a fear of adverse effects and you proceed with medical management. He eventually goes into cardiac arrest and dies, and his family brings a lawsuit against you. What will be the most likely outcome?

A) You are not liable because he refused the treatment that was offered

B) You are not liable because you followed the 'informed consent' standard and documented your conversation with the patient

C) You are liable because patients cannot refuse life saving therapy, and the patient had no real chance of survival without the angiogram

D) You are liable because you did not inform the patient of the risks of forgoing angioplasty

Medical Ethics 101

Answer:

D) You are liable because you did not inform the patient of the risks of forgoing angioplasty

Explanation:

Nowhere in your conversation did you inform the patient of the risks of not having the recommended treatment (angiogram). Since he was not aware that he would likely die without this, he was not fully informed which makes you potentially liable.

For consent to be legitimate, it has to contain the following elements:
- The nature of the procedure
- The most significant risks of the procedure
- The benefits of the procedure
- Any possible alternatives to the procedure, including the risks of not having anything done

Bubb v Brusky, 2009:
Patient was diagnosed with a TIA; his symptoms resolved and a CT scan of his head did not show any acute findings. The physician discussed the case with a neurologist who scheduled close outpatient followup, and he was discharged home. The next day the patient suffered a stroke and filed a lawsuit claiming that the physician did not inform him of the alternative to outpatient management of TIA, including admission, MRI, and possible carotid ultrasound. The patient alleged that he would have stayed had he known that was an option, which would have prevented the stroke. Wisconsin Supreme Court found in his favor, requiring: "any physician who treats a patient to inform the patient about the availability of all alternate, viable medical modes of treatment, including diagnosis, as well as the benefits and risks of such treatment."[59]

Medical Ethics 101

Case:

A patient presents to your clinic for follow up on test results. He receives a new diagnosis of Familial Hypercholesterolemia. The patient has recently become divorced and understands that the disease follows an autosomal dominant pattern of inheritance which places his children at high risk. He refuses to give consent to inform his ex-wife who now has custody of their children. He threatens legal action if you reveal any part of his medical history to his ex-wife. What should you do?

A) Respect the patient's right to confidentiality

B) Ask the health department to inform his ex-wife

C) Seek a court order to inform his ex-wife

D) Inform his ex-wife of the risk to the children

E) Inform the ex-wife's primary care physician so that he can test her for the disease

Medical Ethics 101

Answer:

D) Inform his ex-wife of the risk to the children

Explanation:

The patient's right to confidentiality ends when it comes into conflict with the safety of others. The children have a right to know whether their lives will be adversely affected by the disease. A standard part of the agreement for most divorces is the stipulation that each parent must inform the other parent of health care issues for their children[60,61].

The health department does not notify in cases of genetic diseases. It notifies partners and the population at risk of transmissible diseases such as tuberculosis, HIV, STDs, and food and water-borne illnesses. Simply notifying the wife's physician is inappropriate as the children also need to be tested; in the event that the wife decides to change to a different physician or is unaware of any need to see her physician she might never talk to the one person you communicated with.

The American Medical Association's (AMA) code of ethics emphasizes that physicians should inform all patients who are considering genetic testing of the circumstances under which they would be expected to notify biological relatives of information related to risk of disease[62].

Safer v Estate of Pack:
The court held that a physician's duty to warn might not be fulfilled by telling only the patient, rather – all of those who were potentially at risk of developing the condition. The plaintiff in Safer suffered from multiple colonic polyps and subsequent cancer – a result of a hereditary condition that her father had been treated for when she was a minor. The lawsuit alleged that the disease was hereditary and that the physician had breached duty to inform those who were potentially at risk of developing the condition by only informing the patient[63].

Medical Ethics 101

Case:

You are seeing a 60 year old male in your clinic following an inpatient admission. He has been hospitalized multiple times in the past few months with complicated urinary tract infections, and finally seems to be doing much better. At the outpatient clinic appointment, his wife hands you two tickets to a football game and states 'my husband and I want to thank you for everything...' She informs you that her husband works at the stadium and receives two free tickets to each home game. He adds that the games are boring and he usually sells the tickets, but wanted you to enjoy them. What is the most appropriate response?

A) "Thanks, but it's against my policy to accept expensive gifts"

B) "Thanks – I can't go but my Dad loves football and I'm sure he'll enjoy these...."

C) "Thanks – I'll have fun at the game; but you should know that I give you the same level of care I give all of my patients"

D) "Thanks - I don't normally accept gifts, but since they were free to you I can accept them"

E) "How much do you normally sell them for?"

Answer:

A) "Thanks, but it's against my policy to accept expensive gifts"

Explanation:

The legality of accepting gifts can vary from office to office. Some have a strict policy of never accepting gifts from patients, others set a limit on how much value one can accept from patients. As a general rule, it is permissible to accept small tokens of appreciation – such as a box of cookies for instance. The value for a pair of football tickets should be considered too high – as evidenced by the fact that the patient normally sells them for a profit. The AMA also recommends considering how accepting or rejecting a gift will have a positive or negative impact on the patient-physician relationship[64]. For instance, in some cultures it might be considered customary to express appreciation by gifting a small token. Declining the patient the right to express such gratitude could be insulting and harm your relationship with him.

As a general rule, never accept cash from patients. It should go without saying that gifts should not influence any decisions you make with regards to the care of your patients.

Medical Ethics 101

Case:

A 16 year old female presents to your clinic accompanied by her mother. She has lost weight and her mother admits that she is always complaining of abdominal pain and refusing to eat. She is dizzy upon standing, weak, and orthostatic. After completing your assessment, you suspect that she has anorexia nervosa. You explain to her that she will need hospitalization for IV fluids and treatment. The patient gets very upset, shouting, "You can't do this to me! It's my body and I can do whatever I want!" How should you respond?

A) Encourage the patient to stay for hospitalization, explaining the benefits of treatment

B) Allow the patient to leave, but have her sign an AMA (against medical advice) form

C) Since her mother is her legal guardian, ask the mother to make a decision

D) Speak privately with the mother to ascertain additional information

E) Admit the patient against her will as she lacks capacity

Medical Ethics 101

Answer:

A) Encourage the patient to stay for hospitalization, explaining the benefits of treatment

Explanation:

The patient has put her health in jeopardy – she is dizzy, weak, and orthostatic – allowing her to continue down this road untreated is irresponsible. However, it is difficult to justify keeping the patient against her will. Since her life is not in imminent danger, you can't force treatment upon her. Encouraging her to be hospitalized is the right thing to do, and making sure she is fully informed of all of the benefits of being admitted is appropriate. Speaking privately with either party might provide additional history and can be done at some point, but is not the next most appropriate course of action. Paternalism is when the physician makes a decision regarding what is best for a patient on his own - this is in contrast to autonomy which grants patients the power to make their own decisions.

Medical Ethics 101

Case:

You are a surgeon caring for a 40 year old male who is admitted for abdominal pain. The patient's CT scan shows inflammation surrounding his appendix and you are planning on taking him to the operating room for an appendectomy at the next available opening in the schedule. After informing the patient of your plan, you exit the patient's room and encounter his wife. She asks what has happened to her husband and what is planned. What is the most appropriate course of action?

A) Inform the patient's wife of his condition as she is his legal next of kin

B) Inform the patient's wife that you will need consent from her husband before discussing

C) Inform the patient's wife that her husband has appendicitis, but also tell her that she must discuss any additional details with her husband

D) Inform the patient's wife that her husband has abdominal pain, but do not give any additional information

Medical Ethics 101

Answer:

B) Inform the patient's wife that you will need consent from her husband before discussing

Explanation:

A patient must give consent before any medical information can be disclosed. Sometimes patients don't want other family members to know the details of their care or even the fact that they are in the hospital. Without knowing what sort of relationship the patient and his spouse have, you can't assume that he would want her informed.

HIPAA (Health Insurance Portability and Accountability Act): the first national legislation to assure every patient has protected health information. Hospitals and healthcare workers must inform patients in writing of how their health data will be used, establish systems to track disclosure, and allow patients to review and obtain copies of their own health information. HIPAA made it illegal to disclose a patient's health information to any person who is not a member of the healthcare team.

Medical Ethics 101

Case:

A 76 year old male presents to the emergency department with a headache and fever. After a lumbar puncture, he is diagnosed with meningitis. He refuses antibiotics on the grounds that he and his family have had anaphylactic reactions to several different ones in the past. He is septic and agrees to admission and IV fluid hydration. He later becomes unresponsive and requires resuscitation. What is the best response?

A) Resuscitate the patient to the best of your ability, and start antibiotics

B) Using the principle of substituted judgment, do not resuscitate the patient

C) Attempt to contact his spouse or other members of his family to determine what he would have wanted done

D) Using the principle of implied consent, resuscitate the patient to the best of your ability

E) Using the principle of paternalism, resuscitate the patient to the best of your ability

F) Using the principle of autonomy, do not resuscitate the patient

Medical Ethics 101

Answer:

D) Using the principle of implied consent, resuscitate the patient to the best of your ability

Explanation:

The patient has made clear that he intends to prolong his life. He gives justification for wanting to avoid antibiotics (and presumably understands the risks), while consenting to admission and rehydration. Therefore there is no indication that the patient wishes to have a 'do not resuscitate' order. While the patient will likely require antibiotics, without knowing more information about what may or may not be in his allergy profile it is difficult to start them empirically. Indeed, if he was truly allergic to all options, then he may require desensitization or prophylactic therapy for anaphylaxis. Given the urgency of his situation, attempting to contact family members to obtain consent is inappropriate.

In this case, implied consent refers to a situation wherein the legal requirement to obtain consent is outweighed by the need to render emergency medical care without the patient's consent. The law assumes that an unconscious patient would consent to emergency care if the patient were conscious and able to consent.

Medical Ethics 101

Case:

You are caring for an inpatient male infant who was born premature. He is underdeveloped and now, after several months, is having recurrent kidney stones. His mother insists that you use natural treatments and suggests Pulsatilla flower, which may be of benefit. She finds out you have ordered IV fluids and antibiotics but is upset that you are not encouraging the nurses to use the homeopathic remedies. She questions your credentials and requests that you transfer her son to another hospital. Which of the following is most appropriate?

A) Explain that the Pulsatilla flower can cause vomiting, diarrhea, and convulsions – and is therefore not a recommended treatment

B) Inform the mother that you will order the use of the natural treatment, but in reality continue therapy without it

C) Ensure the mother that you are well-trained and that her child is getting the best care possible

D) Agree on a plan whereby you treat her son's symptoms your way for now, then use the mother's plan once the child is a little more developed and has lower risk for side effects

Medical Ethics 101

Answer:

D) Agree on a plan whereby you treat her son's symptoms your way for now, then use the mother's plan once the child is a little more developed and has lower risk for side effects

Explanation:

In order to be an effective physician, you must be accepting of others' beliefs. Without knowing what kind of background your patients come from, you should not attempt to discredit or devalue their suggestions. So long as there is no harm done to the patient, it is advisable to work together with the family to agree on a plan of care. Never order a treatment without informing the family what you are doing, and never mislead them by giving false information. Emphasizing your credentials is not satisfactory – the mother is not focused on a perceived lack of education in her physician – she is concerned that you are not using her form of therapy.

Medical Ethics 101

Case:

A 75 year old woman is admitted to the hospital following a massive stroke. She was intubated in the emergency department upon arrival for airway protection. She does not possess a living will or advance directive. She has two children – her son, who is the elder, is the first to arrive and informs the physician that he would like a DNR order placed. Next, the woman's daughter arrives and claims that her brother isn't interested in helping their mother. He had been the one to encourage the other family members to put her into a nursing home. She wants everything done to extend her mother's life. The mother was widowed and hadn't specified which of her children was to make decisions on her behalf. You have both siblings meet but they cannot agree. What is the most appropriate course of action?

A) Maintain the DNR order since the first-born child has priority to make decisions in such cases

B) Remove the DNR order in accordance with the daughter's wishes since she is more interested in helping her mother

C) Using the substituted judgment standard, make a decision as to whether or not to maintain a DNR order

D) Consult the ethics committee

Medical Ethics 101

Answer:

D) Consult the ethics committee

Explanation:

In cases where a spouse is not involved, the responsibility for end of life decisions belongs to a patient's children. Unless one is specifically designated as a healthcare proxy by the patient prior to her condition, all of the children carry equal weight in decision making. Using substituted judgment is the proper thing to do, however there is nothing in the stem of the question to indicate what the patient would have wanted. For instance, if they can recall ever watching a television show with their mother, where one of the characters was on a ventilator and she commented how she would never want one herself – that anecdote alone would hold significant weight. Therefore the children should be asked to recollect any such examples if they can – remember, substituted judgment is not asking what you or anyone else would want done, rather what the patient would have wanted if they could make the decision. If an agreement cannot be reached, the ethics committee should be asked to weigh in.

Medical Ethics 101

Case:

An orthopedic surgeon comes to your office as a patient. He has a history of seizures as a child, and has had about one per year since medical school. He is on staff at your hospital and admits that during a recent operation he had a complex partial seizure that lasted thirty seconds. He had a brief alteration in consciousness that went unnoticed and this was the first time it had happened at work. He wants you to start him on antiepileptics as he has never taken them before, and plans to have his wife drive him to work from now on. What should you do?

A) Since you work at the same hospital, you cannot maintain confidentiality; set him up to see a physician at an outside facility

B) Inform his supervisor (hospital administration)

C) Prescribe him anti-epileptics but maintain confidentiality

D) Prescribe him anti-epileptics, and if he has a breakthrough seizure, then you must inform his supervisor

E) Since his seizures are so infrequent, inform him that he will not require medication to manage his condition

Medical Ethics 101

Answer:

B) Inform his supervisor (hospital administration)

Explanation:

Hospitals have well documented policies regarding the 'impaired physician' - one who is unable to fulfill professional responsibilities because of psychiatric illness, alcoholism, or drug dependency. The same principle applies here – you have a physician who cannot safely perform his job without placing his patients and others at undue harm. Imagine if, as an orthopedic surgeon, while operating with a saw he has a seizure and transient loss of consciousness! The protection of patients in the operating room trumps doctor-patient confidentiality. Unless you can guarantee that proper treatment would safely allow the surgeon to practice (for instance if he was a psychiatrist, having a temporary loss of consciousness would not place his patients in any danger) his condition should be disclosed to the hospital[65]. In this case, you should first encourage the surgeon to report himself. If he refuses, you are obligated to go to the hospital administration against his wishes.

Medical Ethics 101

Case:

A 19 year old girl comes to your clinic with a two week history of acne on her face and neck. She appears very upset and cries, "Look at my face! I'm hideous!" What is the most appropriate initial response?

A) "How many hours a week do you spend in the sun and do you use sunscreen?"

B) "I understand that you're upset, but let me assure you, this is something that we can treat."

C) "I understand that you're upset; a rash on the face can be embarrassing."

D) "I can prescribe an ointment to help get rid of the rash – but it will take some time and patience."

E) "Do you have any family history of skin cancer?"

Medical Ethics 101

Answer:

C) "I understand that you're upset, after all - a rash on the face can be embarrassing."

Explanation:

Whenever a patient is upset, the first step in alleviating their concerns or putting their mind at ease is to acknowledge their problem. Sometimes, simply repeating what they've just told you is the best course of action. Asking questions to try to move through a differential diagnosis is important, but not the best place to start. Ensuring the patient that this can be treated is imprudent and not advised, since you don't want to offer false hope.

Medical Ethics 101

Case:

A 30 year old male is diagnosed with tuberculosis. He is an undocumented illegal immigrant who has never seen a physician before as he can not afford to miss time at work. He asks the physician not to report the diagnosis to anyone because he is afraid he will be deported. Which of the following is most appropriate?

A) Do not report the case and have the patient wear a mask at all times

B) Do not report the case as long as the patient agrees to isolate himself while being treated

C) Do not report the case, but contact the patient's family members and work site directly to arrange for evaluation

D) Report the case to the health department only

E) Report the case to the health department to ensure that family members and coworkers are identified and evaluated

F) Report the case to the immigration and naturalization service (INS)

Medical Ethics 101

Answer:

E) Report the case to the health department to ensure that family members and coworkers are identified and evaluated

Explanation:

Failing to report the case unnecessarily puts others at risk. Tuberculosis is a mandatory reportable illness, and all close contacts need to be notified so that they can take proper precautions.

Medical Ethics 101

Case:

A 60 year old patient is admitted for constipation and GI bleeding. CT abdomen/pelvis reveals a large mass. The next step in workup is to perform a colonoscopy and biopsy. While obtaining consent, the patient states, "Please don't tell me what it is – if it's cancer, I don't wanna know..." What is the most appropriate reply?

A) "If you don't want to know the results then there is no reason to do the procedure"

B) "Do you have any family members that you would like to have make health care decisions for you?"

C) "You are competent to make health care decisions so I am legally obligated to inform you of your results"

D) "I will need to get a psychiatrist to evaluate if you are competent to make decisions or not"

E) "Are you having any thoughts of wanting to hurt yourself?"

Medical Ethics 101

Answer:

B) "Do you have any family members that you would like to have make health care decisions for you?"

Explanation:

Just as competent patients have the right to refuse medical care, they also have the right to refuse knowledge of their diagnosis if they so choose. The patient should be aware of the risks of refusing this knowledge and attempts should be made to identify a surrogate decision maker for the patient so that medical care can proceed. In general, your first response should be an open ended question meant to encourage the patient to discuss the reasoning behind his decision. Since this is not an option, the next step is to ask who can make decisions on his behalf for his treatment.

Medical Ethics 101

Case:

You work in a busy urban emergency department when the paramedics bring in a patient who has just finished seizing. You read through his medical records and discover that he has a history of pseudo-seizures and possible malingering. Just then the nurse comes outside of the room to inform you that the patient has started seizing again. You have the nurse give the patient a placebo – as she administers normal saline through his IV you shout "I'm giving you a powerful anti-seizure medication!" The patient stops seizing shortly thereafter. After you leave the room the nurse stops you outside and says, "You can't tell him that!" How should you respond?

A) "Placebos are perfectly legal and I did nothing wrong"

B) "You're right – I'll go in and tell him the truth"

C) "If it hadn't worked, we were ready to treat him with real medication – so he was never really in any danger"

D) "Since he stopped seizing, the placebo helped guide my decision making and was therefore important for me to do"

E) "Since you gave the 'medication' you should be the one to tell him"

Medical Ethics 101

Answer:

B) "You're right – I'll go in and tell him the truth"

Explanation:

Placebo medications work by manipulating a patient's expectations – in other words, use of a placebo is equivalent to deliberately misleading a patient. This undermines the principle of 'informed consent'. Patients have a right to know which medications they are being given, the risk/benefit of a specific therapy, and possess the right to refuse treatment so long as they have decision-making capacity. The AMA agrees: "The use of a placebo without the patient's knowledge may undermine trust, compromise the patient-physician relationship, and result in medical harm to the patient..."[66]

Medical Ethics 101

Case:

You admit a 76 year old male with pneumonia. His past medical history is significant for coronary artery disease, diabetes, and hypertension. He admits to smoking a pack of cigarettes daily. You start treatment with antibiotics and inhalers. Which is the most important topic to discuss with the patient at this time?

A) Education about quitting smoking to lessen the chance of dying from heart or lung disease

B) Ask about an advance directive and the patient's wishes for end of life care

C) Education about the need to exercise to improve hearth health

D) Ask about a will so that if something happens during the hospitalization, his affairs are in order

E) Ensure the patient has refills so that he is compliant with his medications when discharged

Medical Ethics 101

Answer:

B) Ask about an advance directive and the patient's wishes for end of life care

Explanation:

All of the other issues are non-acute and therefore non-essential to discuss during the admission process. All patients, when admitted, should be asked about advanced planning and the presence of an advance directive. There is no way to predict what will happen during a patient's hospitalization, and now is the time to clarify what he or she would want done should the need to make decisions arise.

Medical Ethics 101

Case:

There are two patients who are both in need of a kidney transplant. An acceptable donor is received and both patients are an HLA match. Both are on dialysis due to complications of diabetes and are of similar age. One patient had a 45 pack year history of tobacco abuse but has now quit – he has been on the list awaiting a transplant for six months. The other has never smoked before and has been on the list for four months. What is the best justification for who should receive the transplant?

A) The first patient, because he has been on the list longer

B) The second patient, because he did not contribute to his kidney disease by smoking

C) Whichever patient will have a greater improvement in quality of life

D) Whichever patient will contribute more to society by prolonging their life

Medical Ethics 101

Answer:

A) The first patient, because he has been on the list longer

Explanation:

Since 1987, the United Network for Organ Sharing (UNOS) has served as the Organ Procurement and Transplantation Network for the United States. When considering *renal* recipient candidates, the first thing taken into consideration, to minimize the risk of graft refection, is ABO compatibility. Within the appropriate blood type, a formula has been designed which assigns points according to five criteria: quality of HLA matching (maximum 10 points); the level of panel reactive antibodies (either 0 or 4 points); time on the waiting list; age (1-2 points for children < 11 years) and in certain circumstances medical urgency.

UNOS policy does not mention improvement in quality of life as a criterion in selecting organ recipients. In most cases, transplant candidates who would have little improvement in quality of life have a very low likelihood of benefit and would rarely make it onto a waiting list.

The UNOS Ethics Council has stated that, all other things being equal, preference for patients who have waited the longest is a requirement for fairness: "the fair or just thing to do in allocating among medically similar patients is to give the organ to the one waiting the longest."

Medical Ethics 101

Case:

A previously healthy 45 year old male had a sudden onset generalized headache. He lost consciousness and collapsed shortly thereafter. On arrival to the emergency department he is unresponsive – CT scan shows a large intracranial bleed and he is presumed to have a subarachnoid hemorrhage from a ruptured berry aneurysm. He quickly goes into cardiac arrest and is pronounced dead. His wife and two children arrive at the hospital – when offered an autopsy on her husband's body, the wife replies, "I don't know what to do...." What is the most appropriate response?

A) Attempt to contact his parents for consent

B) Have the organ donation network discuss options with the wife

C) Perform genetic testing on a postmortem blood sample

D) Contact the medical examiner to perform a mandated autopsy

Medical Ethics 101

Answer:

D) Contact the medical examiner to perform a mandated autopsy

Explanation:

The law requires that a medical examiner investigate any death occurring suddenly and unexpectedly or from an unexplained cause. This includes deaths of individuals who are found dead without obvious cause, and medically unexpected deaths which occur during the course of medical treatment or during the course of therapeutic or diagnostic medical procedures. Medical examiner autopsies assist in determining cause and manner of death. Permission of the next-of-kin is not required.

Under normal circumstances, a wife's consent takes precedence over that of the parents. Contacting the organ donation network is inappropriate as you need to identify a cause of death – for instance, since infection (mycotic aneurysm) is in the differential, this would need to be ruled out prior to any consideration for organ donation.

Medical Ethics 101

Case:

A 50 year old woman presents to your clinic and admits that her spouse regularly abuses her both physically and emotionally. She is well known to you and has a long-standing history of chronic alcohol abuse. Which of the following is the most appropriate initial response by the physician?

A) "Abuse will only get worse with time – for your safety you should leave the relationship"

B) "There may be a correlation between your history of alcoholism and the abuse"

C) "Were you ever abused as a child?"

D) "Do you feel safe at home?"

E) "Do you know why he abuses you?"

Medical Ethics 101

Answer:

D) "Do you feel safe at home?"

Explanation:

While all of the above are good questions to ask, the most important thing to do is to ensure the patient's immediate safety. If she does not have a safe place to stay you can offer her social services or shelters and make an immediate impact on her situation. The remainder of the options, while appropriate, are meant to help her deal with the problem on a longer-term basis.

Medical Ethics 101

Case:

A 30 year old Hindu woman was recently diagnosed with acute leukemia. She insists on seeing a homeopathic traditional healer rather than undergoing chemotherapy. Which of the following responses is most appropriate?

A) "I recommend that you see an oncologist – if you disagree then you should seek treatment elsewhere"

B) "This is a big decision – I'd like to have you see a psychiatrist to make sure you understand everything before making a choice"

C) "I can recommend a traditional homeopathic healer that I've worked with in the past..."

D) "In addition to seeing a traditional healer, I would like you to consider chemotherapy"

E) "Chemotherapy is the only realistic chance you have of treating your leukemia"

Medical Ethics 101

Answer:

D) "In addition to seeing a traditional healer, I would like you to consider chemotherapy"

Explanation:

You should never refuse to see a patient or defer care to another physician unless the case is outside of your expertise. There is no indication that the patient needs to see a psychiatrist, rather, this is a case of differing cultural backgrounds. Recommending a traditional healer and ignoring the suggested chemotherapeutic regimen sends the wrong message to the patient and goes against what you really feel will help the patient. Likewise, ignoring her suggestion will likely lead to noncompliance, mistrust, and a feeling of degradation. The best choice is to incorporate both options so long as the homeopathic treatment does not interfere with the chemotherapy regimen.

Medical Ethics 101

Case:

An unconscious 40 year old male is brought in with a gunshot wound to the abdomen. His blood pressure is 70/p and he will require a blood transfusion to survive. He is wearing a shirt that says "Don't Taze me Bro – I'm a Jehovah's Witness". As you are deciding what to do, his wife arrives and states that it is against their religion to give blood transfusions, and despite the fact that he might die without it, he would not have wanted it. Should you give the transfusion?

A) Yes

B) No

Medical Ethics 101

Answer:

A) Yes

Explanation:

Jehovah's Witnesses don't accept blood transfusions based on the Bible's command to "abstain from blood" - therefore, they do not accept blood in ANY form.

Such patients typically carry identifying cards or something else to verify their belief. It's considered general practice to have a card indicating advance directive to refuse blood. Since there is no way to confirm with the patient, there are countless possibilities that should dissuade you from just obeying the spouse and withholding lifesaving treatment – they may be going through divorce, she may want to see her spouse dead, she may even be the one who shot him, etc.

Medical Ethics 101

Case:

A 25 year old patient comes to see you in the clinic. She has had several positive home pregnancy tests which are confirmed by a urine dipstick in your office. She admits to being intoxicated and having unprotected intercourse with her husband two months ago. She is still in school and not ready to start having a family. She asks if you can recommend a doctor for her to see about an abortion. She admits that her husband drove her today, is in the waiting room, and is ecstatic at the prospect of being a father. He is absolutely opposed to her having an abortion. What is your legal obligation?

A) None – you don't have to discuss anything with the husband.

B) You must inform both the husband and the wife of the risks of an abortion, and allow them to make a decision together. Ultimately, the decision belongs to the wife.

C) You must inform both the husband and the wife, and if she still wants to proceed he may obtain a court order to prevent the abortion.

D) Find out more about why she wants the abortion, and try to convince her otherwise.

Medical Ethics 101

Answer:

A) None – you don't have to discuss anything with the husband.

Explanation:

Courts have consistently decided that a woman's right to an abortion can't be vetoed by a husband, partner, or ex-boyfriend, and also that a woman doesn't have to notify the father that she intends to have an abortion.

Planned Parenthood v. Danforth (1976) and Planned Parenthood v. Casey (1992):
Supreme Court ruled that requiring women to notify fathers of abortion placed too great of a burden on women. The Supreme Court ruled: "it cannot be claimed that the father's interest in the fetus' welfare is equal to the mother's protected liberty..."[67]

Medical Ethics 101

Case:

You are a physician attending a fundraiser when one of the wealthy donors goes into cardiac arrest. You start CPR and he regains a pulse before paramedics arrive. His wife is grateful and writes you a check for $500 to cover the cost of your seat at the fundraiser. A few months later you receive a notice in the mail indicating that you are being sued. You are shocked to discover that the man suffered a pneumothorax from your aggressive compressions. Are you liable?

A) No, because he survived and suffered no serious long-term complication

B) No, because you performed to the best of your ability and if you had not intervened, he could have died

C) Yes, because you accepted compensation

D) Yes, because the complication was a direct result of your actions

Medical Ethics 101

Answer:
C) Yes, because you accepted compensation

Explanation:
In most states, accepting compensation or sending a bill complicates the issue of whether you had a pre-existing duty to provide care to the individual, and therefore might revoke your Good Samaritan immunity.

Who is the Good Samaritan?
A man was traveling from Jerusalem to Jericho when robbers attacked him and left him for dead by the side of the road. A priest happened to be traveling the same road, but when he saw the man he passed by on the other side. A Samarian traveler who came upon him cared for his wounds and took the man to an inn. The next day he took out two silver coins and gave them to the inn-keeper saying, "Take care of him. If you spend more than what I have given you, I shall repay you on my way back."

Noble v Sartori (1990):
Two brothers were working together when one developed chest pain and felt like he was having a heart attack. They went to the nearest hospital – a doctor passed by as they were in the waiting room and they asked for help. The physician, who was not on duty at the time, replied, "Get in line and sign in." The physician then walked away. Frustrated, they went to another hospital where he died the next day of an MI. A lawsuit was filed against the physician, who responded by saying that no physician-patient relationship had been formed so he was not liable. The court ruled in favor of the physician: 'although we find [the defendant physician's] callous disregard for the patient to be morally reprehensible, we can find no legal duty to treat a non-patient.'[68]

Medical Ethics 101

Case:

A woman is driving when she observes another car swerve to avoid a deer and go into a ditch. The car rolls over once but lands with the proper side up. The woman stops to help and although there are no immediate signs of danger she notices the driver has a wrist deformity and is therefore unable to get out of the car. The woman climbs into the passenger side and pulls her out. She then calls 911 and paramedics spinally immobilize the patient and take her to the hospital. Later, it is determined that the woman had a cervical spine fracture that became displaced as a result of being pulled out of the car. She is now paralyzed and sues the woman who originally stopped to help her. Is the woman protected under the Good Samaritan law?

A) Yes

B) No

Medical Ethics 101

Answer:

B) No

Explanation:

There was no danger of remaining in the car - Good Samaritan provisions are not universal in application. In the absence of imminent peril, the actions of a rescuer may be perceived by the courts to be reckless and therefore not deserving of legal protection. In this case the intentions were good, but the court can rule that Good Samaritan laws do not apply because the victim was not in imminent peril and hold the actions of the rescuer to be unnecessary and reckless.

Three sample cases with different outcomes:
1. Displacing a cervical spine fracture in the ER: malpractice
2. Displacing a cervical spine fracture in a roadside accident where there was no harm in leaving the patient in the car: likely malpractice
3. Displacing a cervical spine fracture in a roadside accident where the patient *was* in imminent danger: protected

Medical Ethics 101

Case:

A 65 year old man suffered a stroke three months ago. He has persistent right sided weakness as a result. He is at increased risk for which of the following?

A) Major depressive disorder

B) Obsessive-compulsive disorder

C) Post traumatic stress disorder

D) Antisocial personality disorder

E) Social phobia

F) Agoraphobia

Medical Ethics 101

Answer:

A) Major depressive disorder

Explanation:

Major depressive disorder is considered the most frequent and important psychiatric consequence of stroke. As many as 33% of stroke survivors experience major depression, and this tends to peak 3-6 months after stroke. Almost 50% of cases resolve within the first year. The higher the severity of stroke (ie loss of activities of daily living), the higher the incidence of depression[69].

Medical Ethics 101

Case:

One of your colleagues is out of town so you are covering for his patients. A patient presents with low back pain. In his chart, you see that he has received x-rays, an MRI, and has been treated with several different pain medications unsuccessfully. He has asked for referral to a neurosurgeon, despite negative imaging, to see if anything else can be done – but his doctor has held off on doing so. The patient appreciates you giving him a refill of naproxen, but starts to talk about how he doesn't trust his regular doctor and doesn't think he is a qualified physician. What should be your response?

A) Notify your colleague after the patient has left

B) Advise the patient to notify his doctor of his concerns

C) Advise the patient to establish care with a new doctor

D) Inform the patient how to properly file a complaint so that his concerns can be addressed

Medical Ethics 101

Answer:

B) Advise the patient to notify his doctor of his concerns

Explanation:

The best first step is to encourage the patient to bring up his concerns with his regular doctor. If still unsatisfied, he can file a complaint or choose to see a different doctor – but you should always encourage open communication as a first resort.

Medical Ethics 101

Case:

75 year old male presents to the ER in respiratory distress and unable to answer questions. According to his chart he has a history of metastatic lung cancer for which he recently completed chemotherapy. He does not have an advance directive or living will. His wife and son are also present and request that you not intubate him as his cancer is so advanced and he has 'lived a full life and does not need to suffer any more'. What should you do?

A) Intubate the patient anyway

B) Respect the family's wishes and treat him as much as possible short of placing him on a ventilator

C) Ask the family to put their interests aside and think about what the patient would have wanted

D) Contact the patient's primary care physician and see if he has ever communicated his end-of-life wishes to him

E) Obtain a stat ethics committee consultation

Medical Ethics 101

Answer:

C) Ask the family to put their interests aside and think about what the patient would have wanted

Explanation:

Respect for patient autonomy is the dominant principle in medical ethics. In the hierarchy of decision making, the advance directive is the first thing to take into consideration. Substituted judgment is the second line approach, but it's important to determine if the person making the decisions is putting the patient's interests first. In this case, the patient has completed chemotherapy which demonstrates an interest in being treated – had the patient suffered from end stage cancer and been refusing all forms of therapy, that should make you reconsider the decision to intubate. Moreover, the family clearly states 'we don't think he would want to suffer any more' – there is never any indication that the patient himself had expressed these wishes. The third approach to use is that of 'best interest' – which has several limitations and in this case is difficult to determine. In cases of emergency, it's always best to treat first and ask questions later, because it's much harder to question now and treat later.

A surrogate decision maker should attempt to establish (with as much accuracy as possible) what decision the patient would have made if the patient were able to do so. This can be based on previous statements expressed or the surrogate's knowledge of the patient's values, beliefs, personality, and prior lifestyle. Surrogacy seeks to preserve the patient's right of self-determination by placing the patient's own preferences at the center of the decision.

Medical Ethics 101

Case:

A 10 year old girl is brought to the emergency room for a foot infection – she will require IV antibiotics and debridement or is at risk for amputation. Her mother is at the bedside and declines antibiotics on the grounds that she has several allergies to different medications, as does her daughter, and she is concerned that her daughter will develop an allergic reaction. She will consent to the debridement however. Which of the following is the most appropriate course of action?

A) Perform the debridement and withhold antibiotics unless the infection worsens

B) Perform the debridement and administer antibiotics contrary to the mother's wishes

C) Ask the patient if she will consent for antibiotics

D) Refuse to perform the debridement unless you can also administer antibiotics, as the one treatment is ineffective without the other

Medical Ethics 101

Answer:

B) Perform the debridement and administer antibiotics contrary to the mother's wishes

Explanation:

In all situations involving life or limb-threatening cases in minors, physicians may treat without consent. Performing only the debridement and waiting to see if the infection worsens is incorrect and medically negligent. In this case obtaining consent from the patient or one parent is unnecessary. Consent from one parent is adequate and if this were not a life or limb threatening case, this could be correct – however there is no indication that the father is at the bedside or readily available so it is imprudent to attempt to contact him – you should treat irrespective of consent.

Medical Ethics 101

Case:

An 80 year old male presents in respiratory distress from end stage COPD. You decide that he will require intubation. While preparing your equipment, his wife and son arrive and inform you that he does not have an advance directive or living will, but that 'he would not have wanted to be hooked up to machines'. The patient is unable to appreciate the situation and therefore cannot offer much perspective one way or the other. What is the most appropriate course of action?

A) Intubate the patient under the principle of 'substituted judgment'

B) Do not intubate the patient, but admit him to the hospital and make his status do-not-resuscitate (DNR)

C) Do not intubate the patient, and inform the family that he will likely die without this; admit him to the hospital

Medical Ethics 101

Answer:

C) Do not intubate the patient, and inform the family that he will likely die without this; admit him to the hospital

Explanation:

Without an advance directive or living will, spouse and then children should use the principle of substituted judgment to determine how to proceed. In this case, it is reasonable to see how the patient would not have wanted to be intubated so the proper thing to do is to keep him comfortable. There is no indication that he requires a DNR status however. Nowhere in your conversation with the family did you discuss administering antiarrythmic drugs or cardiopulmonary resuscitation (CPR) – therefore, should he go into cardiac arrest it would still be proper to use such measures. The next step in care is to clarify these issues.

Medical Ethics 101

Case:

A patient presents to the ER following an allergic reaction to shrimp. He is in distress and will need intubation. Although he is currently protecting his airway and able to speak, his tongue is swollen and seems to be even moreso compared to when you first saw him fifteen minutes ago. Under normal circumstances you would intubate the patient – however he has a history of being intubated last year following angioedema secondary to ACE inhibitor use. He had a prolonged course and ended up receiving a tracheotomy – after which he was so put off by the whole thing that he had an advance directive made outlining that under no circumstance would he want to be intubated again. When the nurses are out of the room gathering medications, and you are alone with the patient, he is able to tell you in gasped breaths, 'Doc, I decided I want the tube again. I've changed my mind about that whole advance directive thing.' What should you do?

A) Respect the advance directive and treat him with everything short of intubation

B) Attempt to contact family members to determine what the patient would have wanted done

C) Reject the advance directive and intubate if necessary

D) Have him sign a form indicating that he revokes his advance directive

Medical Ethics 101

Answer:

C) Reject the advance directive and intubate if necessary

Explanation:

Advance directives only apply if a patient is unable to make personal medical decisions. As long as the patient remains able to participate in medical decisions, an advance directive can be revoked, and informed decisions by competent patients always supersede any written directive.

Medical Ethics 101

Case:

A 60 year old male is in the preoperative area. He has a history of advanced COPD, diabetes, and hypertension, and has been admitted for a mass that was found by colonoscopy. He is about to undergo a partial colectomy despite being considered a high-risk surgical candidate. After discussing his diagnosis and the planned treatment, the patient admits that he is afraid something may go wrong during the surgery and asks that you pray for him. He has very different religious beliefs than you, and you are not sure how to respond. What is the most appropriate thing to say?

A) "I will be happy to call a chaplain for you"

B) "I am not religious but I will pray for you if you think it will be helpful"

C) "I will be happy to, but just so that you know, my beliefs are different from yours"

D) "I understand your beliefs are very important, and I will keep you in my thoughts"

Medical Ethics 101

Answer:

D) "I understand your beliefs are very important, and I will keep you in my thoughts"

Explanation:

Physicians should at least agree in a generic sense to keep the patient in their thoughts and prayers – this will make patients feel more comfortable, might help place their mind at ease, and improve your patient-physician relationship. Deferring to a chaplain may defeat the purpose – if the patient is more comfortable with you and will feel stronger knowing he is in your thoughts, don't abandon him. Offering the services of a chaplain is certainly important but do not dismiss the patient's request for you to be the one praying for him.

Medical Ethics 101

Case:

You are seeing a 15 year old male in the clinic. He has a history of seizures and has been prescribed phenytoin for management. You check a blood level which comes back low, and you suspect that he has been noncompliant. After informing the patient that his phenytoin level is low, which of the following questions is most appropriate?

A) "How often do you miss taking a dose?"

B) "Taking phenytoin every day can be difficult - what's it like for you?"

C) "In my experience, a low level is usually an indication that patients have trouble taking their medicine as prescribed – do you have this problem?"

D) "If, for some reason, you're having trouble taking your medicine, we can have one of your parents manage it for you to make sure that you take it every day"

E) "You seem to have missed a few doses – do you understand the importance of taking it?"

F) "Phenytoin can have a lot of side effects, but if you don't take it you can have another seizure, which would be much worse"

Medical Ethics 101

Answer:

B) "Taking phenytoin every day can be difficult – what's it like for you?"

Explanation:

There are a few simple rules to follow for most ethics questions. The first is to never assume a patient is noncompliant. Whether it's an insulin-dependent diabetic whose sugar is high or it's an epileptic teenager whose phenytoin level is low – there are a myriad of factors which could lead you to falsely accusing a patient of noncompliance. Chronic alcoholism, use of certain antibiotics, and high doses of salicylate are only a few of those which can lower phenytoin levels. Giving up on a patient for noncompliance before allowing him to explain himself is inappropriate.

Taking control away from the patient and giving it to his or her parents will only antagonize your relationship. Teenagers often battle for control and cherish the opportunity to make decisions for themselves. Taking that away only increases the chances of noncompliance and also has an underlying tone of mistrust. Finally, scaring a patient into taking medication is never the right answer.

Medical Ethics 101

Case:

A patient is admitted to the hospital overnight for unstable angina. Despite it being an academic/teaching hospital, the patient states that he does not want any students taking care of him. The resident does not have time to see all of the patients on his own so he assigns this one to a medical student named Bob Johnson. How should the student introduce himself to the patient?

A) "Hi, I'm Dr. Johnson..."

B) "Hi, I'm Bob..."

C) "Hi, I'm Bob Johnson and I'm a medical student..."

D) "Hi, I'm Bob Johnson, soon-to-be *Dr.* Bob Johnson..."

Medical Ethics 101

Answer:

C) "Hi, I'm Bob Johnson and I'm a medical student…"

Explanation:

A patient has the right to know exactly who is interviewing him about his medical history, performing a physical examination on him, and having input into his medical decision-making. Healthcare workers should never misrepresent themselves and although the medical student has committed a significant amount of time and energy into achieving his or her degree, until they are graduates of medical school they are not technically considered 'doctors'. Some would argue that by coming to a teaching hospital, patients have given 'implied consent' to allow trainees to care for them. Implied consent only applies to emergency situations. Moreover, a patient can always refuse to have a medical student perform any procedure – regardless of whether they are in an academic teaching hospital or not. Of note, students are allowed to perform procedures under appropriate supervision if the patient consents[70,71].

When rounding as a team, attending physicians should first introduce themselves and other members of the team to the patient – explaining each person's role.

Medical Ethics 101

Case:

A 25 year old female is brought to the emergency room accompanied by police officers. She was the restrained driver in a motor vehicle accident earlier, but has no medical complaints. She smells of alcohol and admits to drinking tonight. She is alert and oriented. The police officer requests that you draw a blood alcohol level but the patient does not want this done. What is the most appropriate action?

A) Order the nurse to draw the blood and send it to the lab

B) Order the nurse to draw the blood but inform the officer that you cannot send it to the lab without the patient's consent

C) Refuse to draw the blood without consent from the patient

D) Explain to the officer that blood alcohol levels are notoriously unreliable, and cannot be used alone to convict someone

Medical Ethics 101

Answer:

C) Refuse to draw the blood without consent from the patient

Explanation:

Laws vary state to state, and this is an issue that is always changing. From an ethical standpoint, you should never perform a test on an oriented patient without their consent. This particular blood test is not being used to help or treat a patient in any way.

The Fourth Amendment to the Constitution states: 'The right of the people to be secure in their persons, houses, papers, and effects, against unreasonable searches and seizures, shall not be violated...'

Eckert v City of Deming:
Eckert was pulled over after a traffic violation and was noted to be clenching his buttocks. Police officers suspected that he was hiding drugs in his rectum so a warrant was prepared and he was taken to the hospital for exploration. The first physician refused to treat as the patient refused to consent. Officers went to a second hospital where the patient underwent x-rays, three enemas, and a colonoscopy: all against his will. He sued and was awarded $1.6 million[72].

Medical Ethics 101

Case:

A 22 year old male who plays quarterback for the college football team presents to your clinic for sore throat. He has a high fever, tonsillar exudate, and cervical lymphadenopathy. After drawing some blood, you diagnose him with infectious mononucleosis. After informing him that he will need to avoid all contact sports for the next three weeks, he exclaims, "But the state championship is next week! I gotta play doc!" You inform him that you don't think it's safe, and he replies with a wink, "well, since this is just between you and me, you know, with all that confidentiality stuff, we'll see...." What is the most appropriate response?

A) Document in his chart that you discussed the risks of playing so that you are legally protected

B) Call the student's parents and inform them of his visit and your concerns

C) Call the student's coach and inform him or her of your concerns

D) Re-examine the patient in one week and determine if he is able to play

E) Inform the patient that you used to play football and have a great three point shot – then offer to fill in for him

Medical Ethics 101

Answer:

C) Call the student's coach and inform him or her of your concerns

Explanation:

Most student athletes sign an authorization form that allows information from team doctors or athletic trainers to be shared with coaches. This is meant to protect the patient – athletes with mononucleosis must refrain from physical activity for a minimum of 21 days. At that point a repeat physical examination and possible abdominal ultrasound to assess for splenomegaly can be performed. However it would violate the standard of care to allow a patient to resume athletic activities only one week after being diagnosed.

Medical Ethics 101

Case:

A 40 year old woman presents to the emergency room with constipation. She does not speak English but has her 16 year old son with her. You take a history using her son as an interpreter and it's now time to perform a physical examination. What should you do?

A) Have her son continue to act as a translator

B) Call a hospital translator

C) Ask one of the nurses, who happens to speak the same language, to translate

Medical Ethics 101

Answer:

B) Call a hospital translator

Explanation:

Always use an official translator when possible – this is the only way to ensure that everything you are saying is being communicated to the patient. Family members, regardless of age, might leave out certain details or improperly translate some of the words you are saying, altering their meaning. Also, they will likely not understand the need for word-by-word translation and might cut corners on what they inform the non-English speaker. Using a nurse is also not correct because they may not be able to translate specific medical words which are not typically taught in classes. It is entirely possible to be fully fluent in a language yet not be able to inform a patient of their test results.

Medical Ethics 101

Case:

A six year old child accidentally witnesses his parents having sexual intercourse. The parents are unsure how to explain to the child what happened, and call you for advice. How should you respond?

A) Parents should inform the child that they were just 'wrestling around' and 'play fighting'

B) Parents should inform the child that they were just 'showing each other how much they love one another'

C) Advise them to take the child to a psychiatrist

D) Parents should ask the child what he thinks he saw

E) Parents should avoid talking about it as it is inappropriate for someone his or her age to have to deal with such a sensitive topic

Medical Ethics 101

Answer:

D) Parents should ask the child what he thinks he saw

Explanation:

The appropriate response depends upon the child's development and understanding. The most important thing is for the child to understand that what he saw was not unfriendly or hostile – in other words he needs to know that his parents were not trying to hurt one another. It is also important to get some idea of how the child viewed the incident as this insight can prove valuable to understanding his or her level of comprehension.

In general, if children have been exposed to parental intercourse they need an age-adequate explanation and reassurance about any misconceptions they may have with regards to what they saw.

Medical Ethics 101

Case:

You are eating lunch at a restaurant when a nearby customer slumps over. You rush over to help, and find the person unresponsive. Additionally you note that he has no pulse. You are a family medicine physician and don't typically encounter such emergencies. Nonetheless, you perform CPR to the best of your ability, alternating compressions and rescue breathing at a ratio of 15:2. The paramedics arrive but the patient does not survive. Later, while you are telling your story of heroism, they correct you and note that the new recommendations are to perform this resuscitation at a ratio of 30:2. Are you liable or are you protected under the Good Samaritan law?

A) Liable because you did not follow the standard of care

B) Protected because you acted to the best of your professional ability

C) Protected because if you had done nothing, the patient would have had no chance for survival

Answer:

B) Protected because you acted to the best of your professional ability

Explanation:

Aside from the obvious defense that performing compressions at the proper rate would probably not have changed the outcome, you have not had any reason to take the new basic life support course – and are performing life-saving maneuvers to the best of your ability. Therefore you could expect to be protected by the Good Samaritan law in your state. Good Samaritan laws protect health care providers unless it can be proven that there was a **gross** departure from the normal standard of care or willful wrongdoing on the provider's part.

Ordinary negligence is when an individual fails to act as a reasonable healthcare provider would under certain circumstances (standard of care). *Gross negligence* is when an individual not only fails to follow the standard of care, but his or her actions are malicious (failing to do CPR because you recognize a patient as a known drug dealer)[73].

Gordin v William Beaumont Hospital:
A patient was involved in a motor vehicle accident and taken to the emergency department, where it was determined that the patient would need to go to the operating room. The on-call surgeon was unavailable so another surgeon, who was not officially on call, was contacted and agreed to come to the hospital. He evaluated the patient and the decision was made to operate. The patient eventually went into cardiac arrest and died. The physician used the Good Samaritan defense and won the case – hence the law may even protect physicians who respond to emergencies when not 'on duty'[74].

Medical Ethics 101

Case:

You are seeing a five year old boy in the emergency department after he tripped and fell down some stairs. He has bruises over different parts of his body that appear to be of different ages. He is accompanied by his father, who seems very caring and concerned about the child's injuries. You suspect child abuse based on the pattern of findings and decide to confront the father about your concerns. He is taken aback at the accusation and adamantly denies ever hurting his child. What is the most appropriate course of action?

A) Obtain x-rays and if your workup does not reveal any findings, discharge the patient home with his father

B) Notify child protective services

C) Call the police

D) Speak to the child alone about whether or not someone is abusing him

E) Admit the child to the hospital to remove him from a potentially dangerous environment

Medical Ethics 101

Answer:

B) Notify child protective services

Explanation:

Child abuse is a mandatory reportable offense. Since there is no way to know everything about a home situation, it is always better to err on the side of caution and the law protects you from any potential false allegations that you make. The father may be unaware that his spouse is abusing the child, or an elder sibling is abusing the child – so it is inappropriate to discharge him home. Speaking to the child alone will be important and can be done with the help of a social worker as well, but regardless of what the child tells you, it is still imperative that you involve child protective services. You alone do not have the authority to remove a child from the care of his parents.

Maples v Siddiqui:
Family sued a physician alleging that the physician negligently diagnosed their child's malnutrition as being caused by inadequate parenting skills. After the child was placed in temporary foster care, it was discovered that the child was suffering from malabsorption syndrome and liver cirrhosis. The child was then returned to his parents. The court found in favor of the physician, arguing that good-faith reporting of suspected child abuse or neglect should protect a physician from liability. The court concluded that the legislature granted immunity with the understanding that a physician might be negligent, and that to permit liability would discourage those who suspect child abuse from making a report. The physician therefore had immunity even when there was a failure to diagnose[75].

Medical Ethics 101

Case:

A first year intern is on call overnight for his internal medicine rotation. It's a particularly slow night, so after doing a few admissions and playing a game of table tennis with the other interns on call, he finally finds some time to take a nap. He pager wakes him up at 3am. It's a floor nurse calling to inform him that one of the patient's he is on coverage for is complaining of chest pain. He asks the nurse to give the patient a dose of morphine and to call him back if the pain is unrelieved. The next morning an EKG is done and the patient is found to have an ST segment elevation myocardial infarction (STEMI). Who is most likely to be sued?

A) The intern who was on call

B) The nurse who was caring for the patient

C) The attending physician who is supervising the intern

D) None of the above

Medical Ethics 101

Answer:

A) The intern who was on call

Explanation:

You may have heard the phrase "time is heart" or "time is brain" in cases of either a heart attack or stroke: both diagnoses are time-sensitive and it is of utmost importance to not delay treatment. In such a case, someone is definitely liable to a malpractice claim. The nurse who was caring for the patient did the right thing by alerting the on-call intern. The patient should have been interviewed and decisions regarding EKG, x-ray, lab tests, aspirin, etc should have been made. For years, courts have treated medical residents, even first-year residents, as true physicians when it comes to the professional standard of care in medical malpractice cases. A lack of experience does not lower the standard of care. By the end of 2006, the National Practitioner Data Bank had cataloged more than 1800 residents as having had at least one malpractice claim against them[76].

Lilly v Brink:
In this case the resident diagnosed indigestion and released the patient, who died later that day from a cardiac event. The court determined that the resident used his own discretion in diagnosing, treating, and releasing the patient. The court viewed this performance as equal to that of any fully licensed physician, so the resident should also be treated as one.

Centman v Cobb:
Court found that first-year residents are practitioners of medicine, required to exercise the same standard of skill as a physician with an unlimited license to practice medicine. The court stated that as a health care practitioner, a first-year resident who assumes treatment and care for patients "impliedly contracts that she has the reasonable and ordinary qualifications of her profession and that she will exercise reasonable skill, diligence, and care in treating the patient".

Medical Ethics 101

Case:

You are a cardiologist invited to attend a dinner at a nice steak restaurant. You discover that the evening is being sponsored by a pharmaceutical representative, and the purpose of the dinner is to listen to a presentation on new treatments for hyperlipidemia. You also learn that they will be giving out $300 tablets as an incentive. Which of the following is most appropriate?

A) Decline the invitation to the dinner altogether

B) Go to the restaurant but decline dinner and the tablet gift

C) Go to the dinner but decline the tablet gift

D) Go to the dinner and accept the tablet gift, but do not allow them to influence which medications you prescribe

Medical Ethics 101

Answer:

C) Go to the dinner but decline the tablet gift

Explanation:

It is permissible to attend a lecture and receive dinner for being part of an audience at a presentation. Accepting either cash or items which are worth significant amounts of cash is not ethically upheld.

Medical Ethics 101

Case:

A neurologist is asked to give a grand rounds presentation at an outside hospital. He is researching new treatments for epilepsy, and one of the anti-epileptic companies is sponsoring his presentation and providing him with $2000 compensation. They do not ask for a copy of his slides or have any input into his presentation. What should he do?

A) Decline invitation to give the lecture

B) Give the lecture but decline the money

C) Give the lecture, accept the money, but inform the audience of the compensation

D) Give the lecture and accept the money

E) Give the lecture and accept the money, to be used only towards the research

Medical Ethics 101

Answer:

C) Give the lecture, accept the money, but inform the audience of the compensation

Explanation:

It is permissible to accept compensation as long as you disclose any potential conflicts of interest to the audience. This allows the audience to make a fully informed decision regarding how much credence to give your data. It is important that your presentation be free of bias and that you should maintain control of its content – if you can't ensure this, then you should probably reject the invitation.

Medical Ethics 101

Case:

A deaf patient presents to the emergency department with a sore throat. He is accompanied by his wife who can both hear and perform sign language (ie interpret). The patient does not appear to be in any distress and through the wife you are able to obtain a history. You order a rapid strep test which comes back positive and plan to administer antibiotics and discharge him. He is afebrile and vital signs are normal. Which of the following is most appropriate?

A) Communicate your plan to the patient through his wife

B) Communicate your plan to the patient by writing

C) Wait for a sign language interpreter to come in and serve as your source of communication

D) Speak very slowly and allow him to read your lips, explain your plan, and administer antibiotics

E) Print out the discharge paperwork and give ample time for him to read through that until he sufficiently understands everything that you have done for him

Medical Ethics 101

Answer:

C) Wait for a sign language interpreter to come in and serve as your source of communication

Explanation:

Whenever you encounter a patient who either speaks a different language or uses a different form of communication, as in this case, you must always use a properly licensed interpreter who has both experience and knowledge in working in the medical field. Without any way to verify what his wife has communicated to him, there is no way to obtain an adequate history. Also, one cannot know what kind of relationship he has with his wife and assumptions should never be made. If a sign language interpreter was not available, communicating by writing – while slowing down the process – would be the preferred choice.

Medical Ethics 101

Case:

You are a male physician about to perform a pelvic examination on a 16 year old girl. Her father insists on staying at the bedside throughout the examination. What is the most appropriate response?

A) Pull a curtain in the exam room for the father to stay behind while you do the exam

B) Have another male chaperone in the room and allow her father to wait just outside the door

C) Inform him that her mother can stay at her bedside but not another male

D) Ask the patient – if she refuses to allow him to stay, ask him to leave

E) Allow him to stay since the patient is a minor

Medical Ethics 101

Answer:

D) Ask the patient – if she refuses to allow him to stay, ask him to leave

Explanation:

In all matters dealing with sexuality, patients, regardless of age, have a right to confidentiality. It is the patient's choice whether or not she undergoes the exam, and who will or will not be present in the room when it is done. Whether the family member is a male or female is irrelevant. Having a chaperone present is recommended but ultimately up to the patient.

Regarding the use of a chaperone, the AMA has stated: "From the standpoint of ethics and prudence, the protocol of having chaperones available on a consistent basis for patient examinations is recommended."[80] What makes the most sense is for male and female doctors to ask all patients whether they'd like another person present during an intimate exam. The rationale is twofold: 1 - by having chaperones, patients may feel more comfortable, and 2 - physicians may be protected against claims of sexual harassment.

Medical Ethics 101

Case:

A plastic surgeon is offering his patients referral bonuses. For each person they refer to his clinic, he will reward them with a $50 gift card to a local spa. Which statement best summarizes this practice?

A) Since a patient is profiting from this, and not another physician, this is considered ethical

B) Since patient referrals should only be made confidentially, and rewarding referrals could potentially violate confidentiality, this should be considered unethical

C) Since patients are being rewarded with a gift card, rather than with cash, this should not be considered unethical

D) Since there is a financial incentive being offered, this should be considered unethical

Medical Ethics 101

Answer:

D) Since there is a financial incentive being offered, this should be considered unethical

Explanation:

Patients are certainly in a unique position to offer an informed opinion of their physician, his or her office, and the overall care provided. However, when given a financial incentive the opinion may become skewed. There are no doubt some who would exaggerate the quality of their experience if it meant they could receive a gift card in return. Even though physicians would not be receiving a kickback directly, by gaining new patients they are gaining an opportunity to bill for services that they never would have performed had it not been for the financial incentive – so it is an indirect form of a kickback and therefore unethical.

The AMA has explicitly stated: "Incentives to patients for referrals, then, can have the undesirable effect of interfering with the truthfulness of a patient's recommendation...the profession should discourage incentives for referrals by patients."[79]

Medical Ethics 101

Case:

A 45 year old woman that you recently diagnosed with breast cancer presents to your clinic. She is behind on payment of her medical bills so has not scheduled an appointment with you in several weeks. She requests a copy of all of her medical records so that she can take them to her attorney and determine if there is enough to bring a lawsuit against you for failing to make the diagnosis earlier. You attempt to calm her down but she is verbally abusive and is adamant on getting copies of all of your notes. What is the most appropriate course of action?

A) Have her sign consent and provide her with copies of all imaging studies and lab results

B) Have her sign consent and provide her with a copy of her entire medical chart including your notes

C) Inform her that you do not have to give her a copy of the chart and that her attorney can contact the office's legal department

D) Inform her that you cannot give her a copy of the chart until past money owed has been repaid

E) Do not give her a copy as it can only be used against you to strengthen a potential lawsuit

Medical Ethics 101

Answer:

B) Have her sign consent and provide her with a copy of her entire medical chart including your notes

Explanation:

A medical record can never be withheld from a patient. Consider it the property of the patient and you must surrender a copy any time the patient signs consent. Regardless of what she intends to do with it (establish a new primary care provider, bring litigation against you, etc) – it is her right to have a copy of her entire medical chart. In fact, if another physician were to ask you for a copy of her records, she is the one who would have to provide consent – therefore it would be wise to consider the record the property of the patient.

Medical Ethics 101

Case:

You are an intern on your ICU rotation. You attend a birthday party and see your supervising resident drinking alcohol, while you remain sober knowing that you have to work the next day. The next day, you see the resident at the hospital and rounding on patients. She appears to be fine. What is the best course of action?

A) Inform your attending of what happened the night before and of your concerns

B) Do not inform anyone

C) Discuss your concerns with the resident herself

D) Notify the residency director

Medical Ethics 101

Answer:

B) Do not inform anyone

Explanation:

There is no indication that the resident is an impaired physician. What she chooses to do with her time off is not of anyone's concern, so long as she is not putting anyone else in jeopardy. If she was intoxicated at work then you have a duty to both discuss the issue with her and to notify her residency director. If the resident came in with the smell of alcohol on her breath or appeared intoxicated, you would have a duty to inform the residency director (her superior, not the attending physician). Failing to do so would make you potentially liable for any harm that came to her patients. Even if you discussed your concerns with her and she acknowledged that she had a problem and would take steps to fix it, you would still need to notify the residency director.

Medical Ethics 101

Case:

A 65 year old woman comes to your clinic for exhaustion and fatigue. Her husband died three months ago in a motor vehicle accident while she was a passenger in the car. She admits she sometimes cries for no reason and sometimes hears his voice. What is the most appropriate response?

A) "Do you have flashbacks to the accident or nightmares at night?"

B) "I'm going to give you a medication that will help you feel better and will help you sleep at night."

C) "Do you think about your husband often?"

D) "I'd like to schedule you an appointment with my colleague who can help us understand why you're feeling this way."

E) "I see a lot of patients for depression, so let me assure you that you are not alone."

Medical Ethics 101

Answer:

C) "Do you think about your husband often?"

Explanation:

This is a normal grief reaction, which can last for up to one year. Invite the patient to talk about her feelings.

The American Psychiatric Association (APA) considered changing the definition of depression in the new DSM-5, which would specifically characterize bereavement as a depressive disorder. In removing the 'bereavement exclusion', the DSM-5 would encourage clinicians to diagnose major depression in patients with normal bereavement after only two weeks of mild depressive symptoms - medicalizing normal grief and labeling healthy people with a psychiatric diagnosis.

In May 2012, the APA announced that although the bereavement exclusion will be eliminated from the definition of major depression, a footnote will be added indicating that sadness with some mild depressive symptoms in the face of loss should not necessarily be viewed as major depression.

Medical Ethics 101

Case:

A 30 year old male jumps off of a bridge in an attempt to end his life. He survives, but suffers a pelvic fracture in the process. He is brought in by paramedics and is hypotensive. While the trauma surgeon is informing him of the need to have surgery and attempting to obtain consent, the patient refuses to sign the forms. He understands that he will die without the surgery but does not wish to live any longer and therefore does not wish to undergo surgery. He is willing to stay in the hospital for pain medication however. What is the appropriate course of action?

A) Take the patient to the operating room anyway

B) Obtain a court order to take the patient to the operating room

C) Find out if the patient has a wife or parents who might be able to provide consent

D) Document your conversation with the patient, indicating that he understands and accepts the risks, and admit him to the hospital for pain control

Medical Ethics 101

Answer:

A) Take the patient to the operating room anyway

Explanation:

Suicidal patients lose the right to make medical decisions for themselves, especially in the case of a life-threatening emergency. They are presumed to lack decision-making capacity. In this case, a young patient with a clear indication to undergo surgery should have no delay and should be taken right away. Contacting other family members and obtaining court orders unnecessarily delays the process and is not legally necessary.

Medical Ethics 101

Case:

A 28 year old Somali woman is brought to the clinic by her husband for cough and shortness of breath for 2 days. You (a male) enter the room. The patient appears distant and shy – her husband introduces himself and states that he brought her. He asks "what can you do to help my wife?" For every question that you ask, he answers. The patient herself avoids all eye contact. What is the most appropriate step?

A) Directly ask the patient to describe her symptoms

B) Ask the patient if she wants to have her husband present during the exam

C) Ask the husband to wait outside so you can examine her in private, with a female chaperone present

D) Explain to the husband that the most complete history would come directly from the patient, and question her about her symptoms

Medical Ethics 101

Answer:

C) Ask the husband to wait outside so you can examine her in private, with a female chaperone present

Explanation:

This exonerates the patient from having to have a potentially difficult conversation with her husband. If she would rather that he stay, she can object. It might help if you keep a female nurse with you, so that he doesn't suspect you are wanting to be in the room alone with his wife. This may just be a cultural difference, but you want to ensure there isn't something else that you are missing (for instance domestic violence).

Medical Ethics 101

Case:

A 16 year old female presents to your office for vaginal discharge. The patient admits to recent unprotected sex and after performing a pelvic examination and wet mount, you suspect that she has gonorrhea. What is the most appropriate next step?

A) Treat her infection and have her follow up as needed

B) Ask her to refer her sexual partner so that you can examine him as well. After examining both, decide what the optimal course of treatment would be

C) Treat her infection and discuss the importance of testing for other STDs

D) Notify her parents, but also provide treatment for her infection

Medical Ethics 101

Answer:

C) Treat her infection and discuss the importance of testing for other STDs

Explanation:

The next best step is to test the patient for other potential sexually transmitted diseases. According to the CDC, chlamydia is the most commonly reported STD in the United States while trichomoniasis is the most common STD in sexually active women. Treating the patient's infection is certainly of utmost importance, but it is inappropriate to merely treat her for gonorrhea and send her home without further testing. There is no indication that you need to inform her parents, as minors can receive treatment for sexually transmitted infections without parental consent. Advising the patient to have her partner tested is also advisable, but you would not withhold treatment on the basis that the patient must be present with her partner.

Medical Ethics 101

Case:

A 26 year old woman comes to you (male physician) for nontraumatic back pain. Her exam is unremarkable. You suggest anti-inflammatories and muscle relaxers. As the patient is leaving, she asks if you ever date your patients and if you would agree to see her socially. Which of the following is most appropriate?

A) Do not pursue any social relationship with her, but tell her that you would like to continue being her physician

B) Agree to see her socially as long as she understands that it is separate from the medical relationship

C) Explain that no social relationship is possible as long as she is your patient

D) Refer the patient to a colleague and begin to see her socially

E) Refer the patient to a colleague but still decline to see her socially

Medical Ethics 101

Answer:

A) Do not pursue any social relationship with her, but tell her that you would like to continue being her physician

Explanation:

Agreeing to see a patient socially raises all kinds of moral/ethical issues. Telling her that you can not see her as long as you are her physician leaves the door open, and suggests that if she gets a new physician you will socially see her.

Dupree v Giugliano:
In 2000, Kristin Dupree received treatment for depression and stress from James Giugliano, a licensed family physician. He prescribed antidepressants and referred her to a therapist for counseling. In 2001, they became involved in a sexual relationship, but after nine months they mutually agreed to end the affair. She confessed the adultery to her husband, who subsequently filed for divorce. In 2005 she filed a malpractice lawsuit claiming that the affair was wrong but that she was unable to control herself. An expert witness testified that her romantic feelings were the result of "eroticized transference," a medical phenomenon in which the patient experiences near psychotic attraction to a treating physician, which the patient is powerless to resist. She was awarded more than $500,000[77].

Medical Ethics 101

Case:

A 35 year old male presents to your clinic to follow up on some lab results. He was found to have iron deficiency anemia. He readily admits that he does not eat meat due to religious reasons, and has never felt comfortable swallowing pills so it is difficult to maintain adequate iron levels. What is the next most appropriate question?

A) "If you don't start eating the right things now, you're only going to have more problems later in life."

B) "I can write a note to your religious leader saying that it's medically necessary for you to be exempt from normal dietary restrictions."

C) "Why does your religion prohibit eating meat?"

D) "Would you like information on other things you can eat to keep your iron levels up?"

E) "Whenever something is dangerous to your health, your religion will permit you to make an exception."

F) "If you don't get your levels up, you might need blood transfusions and shots – it would be much easier to try swallowing the pills."

Medical Ethics 101

Answer:

D) "Would you like information on other things you can eat to keep your iron levels up?"

Explanation:

Regardless of your religious beliefs, it's important to always be accepting of others' views. There is no need to question their religion or try to convince them to do things that contradict their particular set of beliefs. Rather, try to work with them to find a solution that will allow them to maintain their values while not jeopardizing their health. Threatening the patient with what may happen to him later in life is inappropriate as it gives the impression that you are offering an ultimatum – contradict your religion or risk your health. It puts the patient in a difficult position and is not the best way to work through this.

Imagine your religion forbids you from doing something, and someone offers to write you a note excusing you. This isn't like missing a day of work!

Asking a patient additional questions about his or her religion is not a bad idea and will strengthen your relationship and level of understanding – but is not the most appropriate question to work towards finding a solution to this particular problem.

Medical Ethics 101

Case:

A 70 year old male is found to have a pulmonary nodule on chest x-ray. Further workup (biopsy, CT scan) reveals metastatic cancer. As you are approaching the room to discuss the findings, the patient's son stops you outside and says "If it's cancer, please don't tell him." What is the most appropriate response?

A) "I'm sorry, I'm required to tell my patients everything"

B) "Talk to me about why you don't want me to tell him"

C) "I need to tell him what we know – if he is okay with it you're more than welcome to come in while I discuss the findings"

D) "Why don't we go into an empty room and I can tell you what we know so far"

Medical Ethics 101

Answer:

B) "Talk to me about why you don't want me to tell him"

Explanation:

Find out what concerns the son has if his father were to find out. Patients have a right to all information regarding their medical care, but you may learn something from the son that will change the way you present the results or deal with the patient's response. For instance, if you learned that the patient may become depressed if his results have come back a certain way, it would certainly make you more aware of the patient's emotional status. If you learned that the patient might become suicidal, 'therapeutic privilege' would allow you to withhold the information.

Medical Ethics 101

Case:

A 65 year old male is hospitalized for weight loss and dysphagia. A new diagnosis of esophageal cancer is reached – after extensive workup it is determined his life expectancy will be about six months. As you enter the room to tell him the news, his family is sitting around his bed. What is the most appropriate response?

A) "I have some bad news to tell you."

B) "The results of your tests are back. Your cancer is very advanced and the results suggest you have about six months left to live."

C) "I have the results of your tests. Would you like your family to stay or would you prefer they stepped out?"

D) "I have the results of your tests. I'd like to discuss them with you privately."

Medical Ethics 101

Answer:

D) "I have the results of your tests. I'd like to discuss them with you privately."

Explanation:

By asking the family to leave, you're absolving the patient of that responsibility. You're preventing him from having to confront his family. If the patient does want his family to stay, he can always override you and invite them to stay, but at least this way he has that option. It's important to emphasize that family support is of utmost importance. With the patient's consent it's always best to deliver bad news in the presence of another close friend or family member.

Medical Ethics 101

Case:

A 75 year old male carries a diagnosis of hepatocellular carcinoma. His disease has progressed to the point where his physician has placed him on the liver transplant list. He has been on the list for six months and has a MELD score of 30. Another patient has been on the transplant list for twelve months and has a MELD score of 20. Assuming they both live in the same geographic area, if an organ becomes available, which patient will have first priority?

A) The first patient because his MELD score is higher

B) The second patient because he has been on the list for a longer period of time

C) The second patient because his MELD score is lower

D) Neither patient is an appropriate candidate

Medical Ethics 101

Answer:

A) The first patient because his MELD score is higher

Explanation:

In an ideal world, every patient with liver disease whose life could be prolonged with a transplant would be able to receive one. Unfortunately, the number of people awaiting a transplant far outweighs the number of organs available. The model for end-stage liver disease (MELD) has proven itself as an excellent predictor of mortality for those on the waiting list. MELD is a numerical scale ranging from 6 (less ill) to 40 (very ill); the individual score determines the urgency of a transplant. The score is based on using the most recent lab results, including a bilirubin level, coagulation panel, and creatinine level. The national average score for a patient undergoing a transplant is 20. Aggregate time on the list (waiting time) is only used as a tie-breaker when two patients have the same MELD score. In other words, when all other things are considered equal, then the amount of time spent on waiting list comes into play.

Medical Ethics 101

Case:

A 16 year old girl comes to your clinic. She is healthy but is unaccompanied by an adult. She requests a prescription for oral contraception. What is the most appropriate response?

A) "I would be happy to discuss this with you. Please have your parents accompany you on the next appointment and we can take it from there"

B) "I will prescribe the oral contraception to you"

C) "I will prescribe the oral contraception to you, but must notify your parents if they should inquire about your visit"

D) "Since you are not sexually active, there is no indication for contraceptives and therefore I can't prescribe them"

Medical Ethics 101

Answer:

B) "I will prescribe the oral contraception to you"

Explanation:

In cases involving contraception, STDs, prenatal care, or substance abuse – it is legal and appropriate to treat while respecting confidentiality even if the patient is under the age of 18. Encouraging her to have open discussion with her parents is also of utmost importance. Finally, having a lengthy discussion with her regarding her reasons for wanting contraception, the risks/benefits of treatment, and the importance of making good life decisions is important as well.

Medical Ethics 101

Case:

A 28 year old woman who is 41 weeks gestation is offered a C-section as the safest method of delivery. Without one, there is a higher likelihood that her fetus will not survive. When presented with the option to have a C-section, she replies, "There's no way you're cutting me open!" You explain your reasons for wanting to do it but she remains adamantly opposed. What is the most appropriate next step?

A) Attempt to obtain consent for the C-section from the father of the baby

B) Inform the patient that she cannot refuse life-saving measures for her unborn fetus, and schedule the C-section

C) Respect her wishes and allow her to refuse C-section

Medical Ethics 101

Answer:

C) Respect her wishes and allow her to refuse C-section

Explanation:

As long as the child is still in the uterus, the mother can accept or refuse whichever treatment she sees fit. She may refuse a C-section even if this will put the unborn fetus' life at risk. The father has no legal right to make a decision on any pregnancy-related issue. Only the mother can sign informed consent during pregnancy.

Medical Ethics 101

Case:

A 65 year old male suffers from chronic kidney disease and receives dialysis three times per week. He has consented to this treatment without objection. After six months, he informs you that he has now changed his mind and would rather die than continue undergoing dialysis. He is not depressed or suicidal. What is the most appropriate response?

A) Stop his dialysis, knowing that he will likely suffer from volume overload and die

B) Given that he has signed consent and will die without the treatment, continue his dialysis

C) Stop his dialysis - if he returns in cardiac arrest, then emergently dialyze him

D) Obtain a psychiatry consult

E) Get a court order to treat him on the basis that he will die without it

Medical Ethics 101

Answer:

A) Stop his dialysis, knowing that he will likely suffer from volume overload and die

Explanation:

Patients have a right to try a certain therapy for a while and then change their mind. So long as they do not appear depressed and are of sound mind, ethics committees and psychiatrists do not need to be involved.

Medical Ethics 101

Case:

A 50 year old male presents to your clinic for routine follow up. At the end of your visit you decide to counsel him on smoking cessation. He has smoked 1 pack per day for the last twenty years. Which of the following statements is most likely to be effective in encouraging the patient to stop smoking?

A) "Smoking can cause many different types of cancer"

B) "Why do you continue to smoke when you know how bad it is for your health?"

C) "Have you ever thought about quitting smoking?"

D) "Instead of spending all that money on cigarettes, you could be donating it to charity. Wouldn't that make you feel happier?"

E) "From electric cigarettes to nicotine patches, there are a lot of options available to help you quit. Is there one in particular that you would like to try?"

Medical Ethics 101

Answer:

C) "Have you ever thought about quitting smoking?"

Explanation:

Asking an open ended question to gauge the level of a patient's interest in quitting is the best place to start. Attempting to scare a patient (whether it's by listing off all of the diseases associated with smoking or by showing pictures of smokers' lungs) is never a very effective method. Making the patient feel guilty about smoking is also not ideal as it does not help start a conversation about the patient's health, which is what should really be at the center of this. Simply naming the different options and asking the patient which one he wants also won't help accomplish your goal, as it does not address the issue of whether or not the patient is interested in quitting in the first place.

Medical Ethics 101

Case:

A patient that you have known and treated for years presents to your clinic. He informs you that he has cheated on his wife and is concerned that he may have contracted a sexually transmitted disease. Cultures are sent and return positive for gonorrhea. After treating the patient, you inform him of the need to tell his wife, who also happens to be your patient and well known to you. He fears that would threaten his marriage. After encouraging him as best as you can to inform his wife, what is the appropriate response?

A) Respect his right to confidentiality

B) Notify the Department of Health

C) Arrange for the wife to have an appointment in your clinic. Test her at that time, and if the results are positive, treat her appropriately.

D) Decline to treat the patient unless he agrees to tell his wife

E) Call his wife to notify her of her husband's results

Medical Ethics 101

Answer:

B) Notify the Department of Health

Explanation:

It is legal to break confidentiality for certain situations, including partner notification for sexually transmitted diseases. The patient's right to confidentiality in such cases is outweighed by the partner's right to safety. The most appropriate way to do this is to notify the Department of Health and allow them to contact all involved parties (including the person your patient contracted the disease from).

Medical Ethics 101

Case:

As you are leaving for work, your neighbor happens to be picking up his newspaper. He stops to say hello, then asks, "I have a question for you: my two year old's come down with a fever. He seems to be acting fine. I gave him some Tylenol and his temperature came down – is there anything else I need to do?" You reassure him that there are lots of viruses going around and as long as he looks okay and his temperature is controlled he should be fine. Later that night, your spouse tells you, "The neighbor called, irate, because they took junior to the hospital and he was diagnosed with bacterial meningitis. Oh, and he says he's going to sue you…" Are you legally responsible?

A) Yes

B) No

Medical Ethics 101

Answer:

B) No

Explanation:

The existence of a physician-patient relationship is a prerequisite to any malpractice claim. Courts have consistently ruled that no physician-patient relationship exists within an informal consultation. In the absence of such a relationship, there is no grounds for malpractice. In this case in particular, you never saw or examined the child, therefore there was certainly never a relationship – and without that there is no duty to treat.

At the same time, consulting with a patient outside the exam room in an informal setting may not necessarily lessen your legal liability. The best course of action is to tell the patient to come to the office the next day or, if the situation seems serious, send the patient to the emergency room. Physicians should be cautious in informal conversations because *some* courts have ruled the conversation can be enough to create a physician-patient relationship in which you can be held liable for a bad outcome.

Medical Ethics 101

Case:

Your brother, who lives just a few miles away, calls you at 7am and informs you that he has run out of his albuterol and can't see his physician for another week. He asks if you can call in a refill for him. You have never seen him as a patient before. He is going to the lake in a few hours and thinks he will need it when he gets there. Can you legally refill it for him?

A) Yes

B) No

Medical Ethics 101

Answer:

A) Yes

Explanation:

The AMA Code of Medical Ethics states: "physicians generally should not treat themselves or members of their immediate families because their professional objectivity may be compromised in those situations."[78] There are numerous reasons your decision-making might be influenced:

- Personal feelings might skew your objectivity
- A desire to avoid necessary but potentially embarrassing questions
- The patient might be hesitant to discuss sensitive information which could be relevant (abdominal pain, pregnant? Chest pain, stress? Sleep disorders, depression?)
- You might over-reach and treat something outside of your scope

Rules can vary state to state, but most state medical boards discourage such prescribing of medications and, if necessary, encourage documentation. Two areas where it may be permissible are in cases of emergencies and in isolated settings where no other qualified physician is readily available. Physicians should not be the primary or regular care providers for their immediate family members, but giving routine care for short-term minor problems may be acceptable.

Medical Ethics 101

Case:

The same brother calls you again – he just came back from his trip and has an appointment with his doctor in two days. He picked up a cough while gone and has used Tylenol #3 elixir in the past which helps. He asks you to write him enough for three doses – a total of 20mL and well below any amount that can cause overdose or significant side effects. He will come by and pick up the prescription from your office. Can you legally prescribe?

A) Yes

B) No

Medical Ethics 101

Answer:

B) No

Explanation:

While rules governing the use of written prescriptions can vary from state to state, with controlled substances the federal government becomes involved. In such cases, a prescriber *must* have a patient-physician relationship, including a written record. Many states further require documenting a medical history and a physical exam before prescribing any controlled substance.

Medical Ethics 101

Case:

A 12 year old child is admitted to the hospital for further workup of extremity pain. His x-ray is concerning for osteosarcoma and a biopsy is done which confirms these findings. After privately informing the parents of the test results, you go into his room to see if his pain is well controlled. He asks if you have the results back and if he will need surgery or if he can go home. What is the most appropriate response?

A) "We don't have the test results back"

B) "We got those results back, but will need to run some additional tests before making a decision"

C) "What have your parents told you?"

D) "You have osteosarcoma, which is a type of cancer in your bone"

E) "I think someone's paging me...I'll be right back"

Medical Ethics 101

Answer:

C) "What have your parents told you?"

Explanation:

So long as the patient is under the age of eighteen (and is not considered a 'mature minor'), only his or her parents/guardians can determine what information is given regarding test results and diagnoses. Ideally you would go into the room, together with the parents, and inform the child of his condition and what the next step in management will be. However, if for whatever reason the parents choose to not inform their child, you must follow suit.

Medical Ethics 101

Case:

Which type of healthcare delivery system encourages physicians to see fewer patients for the same level of compensation?

A) Fee-for-service

B) Discounted fee-for-service

C) Capitation

D) Fixed salary compensation

Medical Ethics 101

Answer:

D) Fixed salary compensation

Explanation:

A 'fixed salary' model indicates that physicians will earn a guaranteed level of compensation regardless of how many patients they see or the extent of workup that is performed on each one.

Fee-for-service models provide physicians with compensation for every service and test they administer. In effect it can encourage physicians to order more tests for higher compensation. A discounted fee-for-service model is one where physicians are paid for every service and test they provide based on a pre-determined discount off the usual price. A capitation system provides physicians with fixed payment per patient, but does not take service into account. It can encourage physicians to take on more patients but potentially provide fewer services.

Medical Ethics 101

Case:

A 35 year old female who has been your patient for several years comes to your clinic. She confides that she and her husband have been unsuccessfully trying to have children for several months now. You decide to refer her to an OB/Gyn to start an infertility workup. Her husband schedules an appointment to see you the next day. He confesses to having had a vasectomy one year before he met his wife and has never told her this before. He is aware of everything you discussed with her on the previous day. What should you do?

A) You have an obligation to inform the wife, as she is also your patient and you are leading her down a potentially expensive and time consuming process of having an unnecessary infertility workup

B) You have no obligation to tell the wife

C) You have no obligation to tell the wife unless her workup is negative, as a means to explain why she might not be able to have children

D) You have an obligation to inform the wife, as this directly impacts the care you give and can be considered part of her 'social/family history'

Medical Ethics 101

Answer:

B) You have no obligation to tell the wife

Explanation:

The patient's wife might legitimately have an undiagnosed cause of infertility, and the husband might actually be fertile – there is no reason to breach confidentiality; in fact, you have a duty to maintain it. There is no mandate or precedent that states one spouse must always be informed of medical care received by the other (unless infectious disease is involved). Therefore you should do the testing, while encouraging the patient to inform his wife.

Medical Ethics 101

Case:

A 25 year old woman brings her two month old baby into your office for routine vaccinations. However, on this visit the mother states that she has recently read some articles questioning the safety of mercury and thimerosal in vaccines, and a possible link with autism. She is unsure if the vaccines are safe for her baby. How should you respond?

A) "There is no study that has shown a link between the mercury/thimerosal in vaccinations and autism or any other problems."

B) "Let's check a mercury and thimerosal level in your child and if they are high we can discuss alternatives."

C) "Can you bring in those articles on your next visit and we can go over them together?"

D) "Some studies have suggested a link but there is no definitive evidence - the American Association of Pediatrics still recommends the vaccinations, and so do I."

E) "While there are reported risks, if we don't administer the vaccines, your child could acquire measles, polio, or hepatitis, amongst others – all of which could be deadly."

F) "I give these to every child – I haven't had problems with any of them yet."

Medical Ethics 101

Answer:

D) "Some studies have suggested a link but there is no definitive evidence - the American Association of Pediatrics still recommends the vaccinations, and so do I."

Explanation:

It is important to acknowledge the mother's viewpoint while at the same time giving sound medical advice. While there have been reported links, all major medical societies still recommend the immunization schedule sponsored by the American Association of Pediatrics (AAP). There have been alternative vaccination schedules that have been proposed, in which the duration between different vaccines is increased so they are spread out over a longer period of time, but none have officially received endorsement. Threatening a mother with all the various diseases that vaccinations offer protection from is not the most effective way to get her to comply. Having her bring in her own articles unnecessarily delays administration of vaccines.

Thimerosal, previously used as a preservative in many recommended childhood vaccines, was removed/reduced to trace amounts in 2001. There has been no recent decrease in autism despite the exclusion of anything more than trace levels of thimerosal from nearly all childhood vaccines – leading many to conclude that data does not support the hypothesis that exposure to thimerosal during childhood is a primary cause of autism.

Medical Ethics 101

Case:

A 65 year old male with a history of congestive heart failure is admitted to the hospital with shortness of breath. The physician writes a standing order for furosemide 80mg every 8 hours. The nurse checks the patient's vital signs and discovers his blood pressure is 90/60mmHg. She does not agree with the order of furosemide, concerned that it will further lower his blood pressure. She is unable to get ahold of the physician to verify the order. Which of the following actions should she take?

A) The nurse should administer the medication

B) The nurse should administer half the dose and then re-evaluate

C) The nurse should not administer the medication, and document her reasons for doing so

D) The nurse should discuss the risks and benefits with the patient before proceeding

Medical Ethics 101

Answer:

C) The nurse should not administer the medication, and document her reasons for doing so

Explanation:

The primary bond between a physician and nurse is a mutual desire to do what is best for the patient. One of the duties in providing reasonable care is fulfilled by a nurse who carries out the orders of the attending physician. When the nurse feels the order may be an error or contrary to customary medical and nursing practice, the physician has an ethical obligation to hear the nurse's concern and explain those orders to the nurse involved. An ethical physician should neither expect nor insist that nurses follow orders contrary to standards of good medical and nursing practice.

In emergencies, when prompt action is necessary and the physician is not immediately available, a nurse may be justified in acting contrary to the physician's standing orders for the safety of the patient.

Medical Ethics 101

Case:

A 24 year old female suffers from psoriasis. When exacerbated, lesions will appear on her face and neck. She is self-conscious about the attention her lesions receive and asks you for the best way to deal with others' reaction. Which of the following is the best response?

A) "Tell people that it is a private issue and they shouldn't look at you any differently"

B) "Wear makeup and long sleeve shirts to try to cover the rash whenever there is a bad outbreak"

C) "Avoid leaving the house as much as possible to avoid such potentially embarrassing situations"

D) "Make sure others know that there is nothing contagious about the rash"

E) "Pretend you don't notice when they are looking at you"

F) "Use this ointment and it will take care of your outbreaks"

G) "Let me refer you to a dermatologist"

Medical Ethics 101

Answer:

D) "Make sure others know that there is nothing contagious about the rash"

Explanation:

Having an open discussion and addressing others' concerns is the fastest and most effective way of dealing with this issue. While referral to a dermatologist may be necessary, it does nothing to deal with the social issues the patient is experiencing. This is clearly causing psychological duress for her, so asking her to pretend that she doesn't notice when others are looking is unreasonable. Don't provide false hope by promising that a medication will take care of a non-curative condition.

It is better to have the patient face the problem than to act like nothing is wrong or to potentially offend people by telling them that it is not their business. Patients should never be encouraged to remain sheltered inside their home.

Medical Ethics 101

Case:

Dave Woodbridge is a physician seeing a male patient named Jeremiah Smith for the first time. How should the physician begin the conversation?

A) Hello Jeremiah, I'm Dr. Woodbridge....

B) Hello Mr. Smith, I'm Dr. Woodbridge...

C) Hello Jeremiah, I'm Dave...

D) Hello, I'm Dr. Woodbridge...

Medical Ethics 101

Answer:

B) Hello Mr. Smith, I'm Dr. Woodbridge...

Explanation:

Communication with patients should be leveling. That is, if the physician expects to be addressed using a title, then the patient should also be addressed with a title.

Patients should always know who's working with them. Several articles have been written addressing physician etiquette and the consensus is that the first time you are meeting a patient, you should introduce yourself as "Dr. X". Once a level of trust has been established there is certainly nothing wrong with being on a first-name basis with the patient.

Medical Ethics 101

Case:

An 80 year old male is admitted to the hospital with a diagnosis of metastatic colon cancer and respiratory failure. Throughout his hospitalization he continues to decline and eventually develops hospital-acquired pneumonia and renal failure. There is a pulmonologist, nephrologist, and critical care physician amongst others caring for him. Each one meets separately with the adult children on their daily rounds to discuss the treatment plan and recommendations. The family grows frustrated with each passing day as his health continues to deteriorate and eventually accuses you of ordering unnecessary treatments and causing more harm then good. Which of the following is most likely responsible for the family's negative perception?

A) Inappropriate consultations/treatment

B) Poor nursing care

C) Poor physician communication

D) Uncertainty over rising medical bills and lack of insurance

E) Fear that the patient would not have wanted this

Medical Ethics 101

Answer:

C) Poor physician communication

Explanation:

When multiple physicians are involved in the care of a patient, it is imperative that they communicate regularly with each other about treatment objectives and goals. This way, a clear plan can be presented to family members so that there are no unanswered questions. There is nothing to suggest the patient is receiving inadequate nursing care. All of the consultations seem appropriate given his multitude of problems. There is no information available regarding the possibility of a living will or what the patient's wishes may have been, nor is there any indication that the family is upset regarding rising costs.

Medical Ethics 101

Case:

A 45 year old male with a history of diabetes and hypertension presents to the office for a routine follow-up. He tells his physician that he's not able to have intercourse with his wife and it is causing strain on their marriage. What is the best response?

A) "Why are you not able to have intercourse?"

B) "Would you like to try a prescription of Viagra?"

C) "Let's order some tests and see what we can do to figure out the problem"

D) "Let's bring your wife in and we can talk about this together"

E) "I'm going to refer you to a marriage counselor"

F) "This is probably a side effect of your medications. Let's make some changes and see if that helps"

Medical Ethics 101

Answer:

A) "Why are you not able to have intercourse?"

Explanation:

The logical first step is to figure out what the patient means when he says he's not able to have intercourse. What if he is unable to have intercourse with his wife because they work conflicting schedules? What if he no longer has interest in intercourse? What if he has suspicion that she is cheating on him? What if he has HIV and hasn't informed anyone? With the information that is given, it is unclear what the problem is, rendering any treatment recommendations ill-informed.

Medical Ethics 101

Case:

A 45 year old suicidal male presents to the ER after cutting his wrists. Paramedics report that there was a large amount of blood on the scene and the patient's arms are now covered in dry blood. Bleeding is controlled but the lacerations are large and should be sutured closed. The patient refuses sutures, stating he understands that without them he is risking poor wound healing and a much larger scar. Which of the following actions is most appropriate?

A) Since the patient is suicidal, he may not refuse medical care

B) Wait until a psychiatric evaluation is completed before making a decision

C) Contact his spouse or next of kin to obtain consent for treatment

D) Obtain a court order for treatment

E) Explain why you want to suture his wounds: if he still refuses, then do not perform closure

Medical Ethics 101

Answer:

E) Explain why you want to suture his wounds: if he still refuses, then do not perform closure

Explanation:

In almost all circumstances, a patient who refuses treatment after a suicide attempt should be given life-saving treatment. In this instance, bleeding is controlled and the risks of not having sutures placed are given in the question stem: the potential for infection and poor cosmesis. Neither of these mandate treatment, leaving the patient within his rights to refuse sutures.

Medical Ethics 101

Case:

A 60 year old unresponsive male presents to the ER with a self-inflicted gunshot wound to the abdomen. As you are about the pick up the phone to notify the on-call trauma surgeon, you look in his records and discover he has a signed and valid DNR on file that indicates he does not want resuscitation, intubation, or any surgical treatment. His blood pressure is 60/20 and he is actively hemorrhaging. What should you do next?

A) Since the patient attempted suicide, he should go to to the OR for potential life-saving treatment

B) Obtain a court order to proceed with surgery

C) Attempt to contact family to find out more about the DNR form and what they think he would want done

D) Since the patient has a signed DNR, he should not go to surgery and should be allowed to die in the ER

E) Contact the psychiatrist to determine competency and how to proceed

Medical Ethics 101

Answer:

A) Since the patient attempted suicide, he should go to to the OR for potential life-saving treatment

Explanation:

Of all the gray areas of medical ethics, this may be the grayest.
The decision to override the DNR request of one who has attempted suicide is a conflict between autonomy and beneficence or non-maleficence. A large percentage of suicide attempts are irrational acts, and at the time of the attempt the individual does not possess full decision-making capacity. Many patients are suffering from a mental illness that impairs judgment. In fact, 90% of suicides are found on postmortem analysis to be associated with depression, substance abuse, or psychosis. The individual who attempts suicide can be assumed to be suffering from a treatable mental illness, and once effective treatment is provided, they may no longer want to die.

The American Society for Bioethics and Humanities has opined that a suicide attempt nullifies a DNR/DNI order such that every effort to prevent death or revive the person should be made. The reasoning is that DNR/DNI orders are intended to remove barriers to natural death -- as in the case of someone for whom a resuscitation attempt would likely not be successful or cause additional harm even if the person survived. However, a suicide attempt is not the expected outcome of a natural aging/dying process. That being said, there is a growing opinion that in the context of advanced illness, especially one that involves physical pain or suffering, suicide could be considered a rational option. Hence the legalization of 'physician-assisted suicide' in Oregon, Washington, and Montana.

For the purpose of test questions, the clinician should do everything necessary to save one's life, including using resuscitation equipment. If the person is later proclaimed brain dead, an existing DNR order may allow the equipment to be disconnected so that a 'natural death' may occur[81,82].

Medical Ethics 101

Case:

A patient is admitted to the hospital with jaundice and a large pancreatic mass that is discovered on CT scan. A biopsy is done which confirms the diagnosis of metastatic pancreatic cancer. As the physician enters the room to tell the patient he cries, "I just know it's bad news!" What is the most appropriate response?

A) "No, it's not that bad…"

B) "Tell me how you feel"

C) "If it is bad, do you still want to know?"

D) "How would you feel if it was bad news?"

E) "Yes, it is bad news"

Medical Ethics 101

Answer:

E) "Yes, it is bad news"

Explanation:

Patients have a right to know their test results – the exception to this rule is 'therapeutic privilege'. If there is significant evidence that a patient will become potentially suicidal upon hearing the news, then it is permissible to withhold informing them. There is nothing in this question to indicate that the patient is considering self-harm. There is certainly no reason to mislead the patient by reassuring them that the results are good.

The patient is anxious about his results and inquiring about his general attitude is awkward and inappropriate.

Medical Ethics 101

Case:

A nurse approaches you and asks for a prescription for phentermine, a well-known weight loss drug. Knowing that it is a stimulant and a controlled substance, you are initially hesitant. She informs you that she has taken it before. She is new to the area but has already scheduled an appointment with her new primary care physician in two weeks. How should you respond?

A) "Have you had any problems with the medication in the past?"

B) "Why haven't you talked to your new physician about this?"

C) "I am not comfortable prescribing this for you since I am not your physician"

D) "It is always unethical to prescribe medications for friends and coworkers"

Medical Ethics 101

Answer:

C) "I am not comfortable prescribing this for you since I am not your physician"

Explanation:

Physicians are commonly approached by coworkers for informal medical care ranging from prescription for antibiotics to prescriptions for controlled substances. Rules can vary from state to state but most medical bards discourage such prescribing of medications and, if necessary, encourage documentation. Two areas where it may be permissible are in cases of emergencies and in isolated settings where no other qualified physician is readily available.

Medical Ethics 101

Case:

Parents of a seven year old boy are at a loss of what to tell their son who blames himself for the death of his younger sister. She was diagnosed with retinoblastoma and ultimately died after a prolonged period of palliative care. He is now constantly sad and repeats over and over "It's all my fault! She died because of me." What is the parents' best response?

A) "Don't worry, things will be okay"

B) "You're such a strong boy"

C) "Your sister was very sick and the sickness made her die"

D) "You have to be strong to help your mother"

E) "Let's get a new pet"

Medical Ethics 101

Answer:

C) "Your sister was very sick and the sickness made her die"

Explanation:

It is essential to talk to the child, ask questions, and most importantly, reassure him that it was not his fault. At this age, the best response is to be concrete and specific about what has happened. Don't try to avoid the subject: encourage the child to ask questions and address his fears. Do not use cliches as you want to make sure the child understands that he is not at fault.

Childrens' understanding of death varies by age. For testing purposes, children understand that death is final by age 6-9.

From age 2-6 children believe that death is temporary and reversible. They may engage in magical thinking that wishes come true and might feel guilty about the loss of a loved one.

Medical Ethics 101

Case:

A patient presents to the emergency department with a chief complaint of vomiting blood. The nurses establish IV access and start administering IV fluids. A naso-gastric tube is placed and a large amount of bright red blood is suctioned out. You suspect that the patient has an active upper GI bleed. The gastroenterologist agrees to see the patient in the ER and would like to do a bedside endoscopy. He asks that you consent the patient for an EGD while he drives in to the hospital. What is the best response?

A) Discuss the risks and benefits with the patient and have them sign the consent form

B) Refuse to obtain consent and ask the gastroenterologist to obtain it once he arrives

C) Consent is unnecessary in this case since it is a life-threatening emergency

D) Have one of the nurses who will assist the gastroenterologist and be in the room for the procedure obtain consent

Medical Ethics 101

Answer:

B) Refuse to obtain consent and ask the gastroenterologist to obtain it once he arrives

Explanation:

How can you (or a nurse) be expected to fully discuss the risks, benefits, and alternatives to doing a procedure that you yourself have likely never performed? The need to obtain a patient's consent before rendering diagnostic testing or treatment has long been recognized by the law. Lack of proper consent (except in cases of emergency) could lead to charges of battery, even in cases when the care rendered meets standards of practice.

According to the AMA, informed consent is a process of communication between a patient and physician in order to agree upon a specific medical intervention. In that process you, as the physician providing or performing the treatment/procedure (not a delegated representative), should disclose and discuss with your patient specifics of the procedure as well as risks and benefits. The "process of communication" cannot be delegated to another physician.

Similarly, the American Academy of Emergency Medicine has published a policy in cases of acute myocardial infarction. They have made it clear that only the interventional cardiologist should obtain informed consent for cardiac catheterization.

Medical Ethics 101

Case:

A mother brings her sixteen year old daughter in to your clinic for a 'regular check up'. You see her and over the course of the next two years continue to be her primary care physician. Eventually she moves away for college. One year later you run into her mother at a coffee shop and she asks you out for dinner. What is the best response?

A) "Yes – since I never saw you as a patient, it is ethically permissible"

B) "Yes – since your daughter is no longer my patient, it is ethically permissible"

C) "No – since your daughter was my patient, it is not ethically permissible"

D) "No – I don't eat dinner"

Medical Ethics 101

Answer:

C) "No – since your daughter was my patient, it is not ethically permissible"

Explanation:

Remember that a physician-patient relationship is permanent. There are instances in which it can be broken, but barring those circumstances that patient should always be considered to be yours. Parents play an integral role in the decision-making process for their underage children (with rare exception they must provide consent for all medical decisions), and should be considered part of the physician-patient relationship.

The American Psychiatric Association makes this very clear, stating: "Romantic involvement either during or subsequent to treatment with key family members may be construed as exploitation of the patient and family...this may discourage the original patient and other family members from seeking subsequent treatment...Romantic involvement with key family members is also unethical."

Medical Ethics 101

Appendix I.
KEY ETHICAL PRINCIPLES:

Autonomy	Respecting a patient's right to make their own decision regarding medical care
Beneficence	Actions done for the benefit of others (CPR, vaccinations, education and counseling)
Non-maleficence	Do no harm (Stopping harmful medications, not prescribing treatments that are ineffective)
Justice	Be as fair as possible when offering treatments to patients and allocating scarce medical resources

Double Effect: Two different types of consequences from one action; usually combined beneficence and non-maleficence (morphine as both an analgesic and a respiratory depressant in a dying patient)

Decision-making capacity: Patients have a right to autonomy even if the decision is unwise. Autonomy is only possible when a patient possesses the ability make decisions; the following are required components:
- Understand the medical diagnosis and prognosis
- Understand the recommendations and alternatives
- Acknowledge the risk and benefit of each alternative
- Using logical reasoning to make a decision
- Decision does not fluctuate and remains stable with time

Medical Ethics 101

<u>Paternalism</u>: Healthcare professionals make decisions for the patient

<u>Therapeutic Privilege</u>: Withholding information when having that information can cause serious psychological harm to a patient

<u>Informed Consent</u> components:
- Full disclosure
- Comprehension on behalf of the patient (capacity)
- Lack of coercion

<u>Implied Consent</u>: Presumed consent obtained when a patient is either unconscious or incompetent or no surrogate decision-maker is present

<u>Good Samaritan</u> requirements:
- True emergency (potential for loss of life or limb)
- No compensation (care is given in good faith)
- No abandonment (once care is commenced you must remain at the scene until someone capable of taking over arrives)
- No gross negligence

<u>Malpractice</u> components; all four are required for a successful claim:
- **D**uty to treat
- **D**eviation from standard of care
- **D**amage to the patient
- **D**amage occurred directly as a result of physician's actions

Medical Ethics 101

Appendix II.
LEARNING AND BEHAVIOR MODIFICATION

In each of the following cases, choose which type of learning and behavior pattern is being demonstrated:

1) A person is attempting to quit smoking cigarettes. He is shown several short videos and each time someone is shown smoking, he receives a small electrical shock.
2) A newborn is thirsty for milk – she reaches for the mother's nipple instinctively.
3) A woman suffers from tension headaches. She is taught different mental relaxation techniques to decrease the tension and treat her headache.
4) A child is being toilet trained. Each time he successfully uses the toilet, he is given one of his toys to play with.
5) A man suffers from high cholesterol. He begins to diet and exercise in order to avoid having to take statin medications.
6) Two children are fighting – the mother sends one to his room and tells him 'go to your room until you apologize!"
7) A mother scolds her young son for spending so much time at the local comic book store. She forbids him from going there after school. As a result, he starts to spend even more time there.
8) Each time a patient comes to see his physician, he is noted to have high blood pressure. But when he checks it on his own at home, it is always normal.

Answer choices (may be used more than once):
A) Operant conditioning
B) Classical conditioning
C) Biofeedback
D) Negative reinforcement
E) Aversive conditioning
F) Positive reinforcement
G) Imprinting

Medical Ethics 101

Answers:
1 – E, 2 – G, 3 – C, 4 – A, 5 – D, 6 – D, 7 – F, 8 – B

Classic conditioning
An unconditioned stimulus and conditioned stimulus are paired
Reflexive natural response occurs because of a learned stimulus
Examples: Pavlov's dog – sound of bell is paired with feeding, so when the bell sounds the dog begins to salivate without even seeing the food; white coat hypertension (pt sees a physician and his blood pressure starts to rise)

Operant conditioning
Learned behavior as a result of rewards or punishments associated with it
Consider positive/negative punishment and positive/negative reinforcement

Positive and Negative Punishment vs Positive and Negative Reinforcement

Punishment: A consequence immediately follows a behavior - which **decreases** the future frequency of that behavior. A stimulus can be added (positive punishment) or removed (negative punishment). The end result is to decrease a behavior.

Positive punishment involves adding a negative consequence after an undesired behavior.
Examples: child punches his brother (behavior) and is sent to his room (consequence), man lies to his physician about medication compliance (behavior) and is fired from seeing that physician (consequence)

Negative punishment involves removing a desired stimulus after an undesired behavior.
Examples: child who enjoys video games (desired stimulus) has them taken away (removed) when he refuses to share (undesired behavior), man who enjoys cocaine (desired stimulus) is put into detox (removed) after his wife discovers he has spent all their savings on it (undesired behavior)

Medical Ethics 101

Reinforcement: A stimulus immediately follows a behavior – which **increases** the future frequency of a specific behavior. The end result is to increase a behavior.

Positive reinforcement works by adding a stimulus that will motivate the individual to repeat a desired behavior.
Examples: giving a child a token (stimulus) each time he brushes his teeth (desired behavior), rewarding patients with money (stimulus) for losing weight (desired behavior)
Mother scolds a child for going to the comic book store (stimulus) – now the child goes even more (behavior). In this case, even though it is a behavior that might not be thought of as 'positive', the stimulus increased the behavior.
A child cries about not getting dessert after dinner, so the parents give it to him. Now the child cries after dinner every night.

Negative reinforcement occurs when a particular behavior is exhibited to remove a certain stimulus (usually an aversive one). Again, you are attempting to increase a behavior.
Examples: husband mowing the lawn (behavior) to avoid having his wife nag (to remove stimulus), patient taking his medications (behavior) to avoid embarrassment of admitting noncompliance to his physician (to remove stimulus)
Two brothers are fighting – the mother says 'go to your room until you apologize' – the mother is attempting to increase a behavior (apologize) by removing a stimulus (sending child to his room)

Imprinting
One acquires attachment to another simply by being associated
Examples: birds learning how to fly or babies knowing how to feed

Shaping
Successive behavior is rewarded until the complete behavior is demonstrated
Example: toilet training

Medical Ethics 101

Extinction
Behavior becomes less frequent and weaker when it is no longer reinforced
Example: child goes to the nurse's office everyday so eventually she stops taking him seriously (the unwanted behavior will eventually stop); leaving a child in 'time out' when they begin to cry halfway through

Systematic desensitization
Behavioral modification based on classical conditioning
Example: person is scared of heights so they start low and slowly get higher and higher until they conquer their fear

Exposure
Forced exposure to until a response is eliminated
Example: person is scared of spiders so they are put in a room full of spiders
Also known as 'flooding' or 'implosion' in extreme cases

Fading
Removing a stimulus slowly to remove a particular behavior
Example: lowering the alcohol content of each drink a person takes until they cannot notice that there is no alcohol in their drink

Biofeedback
Modifying autonomic nervous system responses (blood pressure, heart rate, etc) through external stimuli
Example: listening to music therapy to treat migraine headaches

Aversive conditioning
Making something less desirable (aversive)
Example: patient who wishes to stop consuming alcohol is given disulfiram which causes vomiting when taken concomitantly with alcohol

Medical Ethics 101

INDEX

Topic	Page Numbers
Autonomy	15, 37, 77, 91, 95, 107, 133, 143, 197, 229
Informed Consent	13, 23, 31, 39, 41, 77, 85, 121, 123, 147, 177, 195, 237
Consent for Minors	9, 25, 39, 49, 57, 71, 81, 91, 135, 167, 181, 193, 209
Confidentiality	11, 19, 59, 63, 69, 73, 83, 87, 93, 101, 123, 149, 179, 181, 187, 189, 193, 201, 209, 213
Depression	7, 81, 129, 175, 177, 227, 229
Therapeutic Privilege	17, 107, 187, 231
Communication	43, 45, 47, 65, 79, 83, 103, 107, 109, 111, 117, 119, 131, 141, 143, 145, 151, 153, 165, 179, 185, 189, 199, 203, 209, 215, 217, 219, 221, 223, 231, 235
End-of-life Issues	15, 29, 33, 95, 99, 111, 133, 137, 139, 197, 229
Abortion	37, 57, 123
Organ Donation	21, 27, 35, 55, 75, 113, 115, 191
Good Samaritan	125, 127, 155, 203
Communicable Diseases	45, 47, 53, 61, 63, 105, 181, 201
Child Abuse	79, 157
Doctor & Patient	17, 61, 67, 69, 89, 97, 109, 119, 131, 141, 145, 183, 221, 225, 239
Doctor & Society	11, 19, 67, 73, 161, 203, 205, 207, 211, 233
Doctor & Doctor	51, 131, 169, 173, 223, 237
Malpractice	61, 85, 159, 171, 205, 207

Medical Ethics 101

Medical Ethics 101

*If you have questions, comments, or would like to share your text experience, please feel free to email the authors at **ultimateEMguide@gmail.com***

*For a complete list of references from the book or to read about more interesting cases, please visit the author's website at **www.myERdoctor.com***

Made in the USA
Columbia, SC
26 August 2018